SOFT TISSUE RELEASE

A PRACTICAL HANDBOOK FOR

PHYSICAL THERAPISTS

SOFT TISSUE RELEASE

A PRACTICAL HANDBOOK FOR

PHYSICAL THERAPISTS

Mary Sanderson

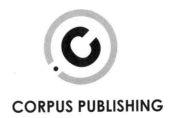

CORPUS PUBLISHING

© Corpus Publishing Limited 2002

First published in 1998 by Otter Publications (ISBN 1 899053 12 3 and reprinted by Corpus Publishing Limited ISBN 1 903333 00 8).

This new edition published in 2002 by
Corpus Publishing Limited
PO Box 8, Lydney, Gloucestershire, GL15 4YN.

Author's notes
Though the photographs show both male and female subjects, I refer to 'he' throughout this book for the sake of grammatical consistency.

Disclaimer
This publication is intended as an informational guide. The techniques described are a supplement, and not a substitute for, professional medical advice or treatment. They should not be used to treat a serious ailment without prior consultation with a qualified healthcare practitioner. Whilst the information herein is supplied in good faith, no responsibility is taken by either the publisher or the author for any damage, injury or loss, however caused, which may arise from the use of the information provided.

British Library Cataloguing in Publication Data
A CIP record for this book is available from the British Library
ISBN 1903333 09 1

Acknowledgements
I would like to thank the London School of Sports Massage for introducing me to such a satisfying and inspiring career, and to my colleagues there for encouraging me to write about STR. I also wish to thank Mel Cash, Graham Anderson, John Sharkey, Chris Salvary, Tanya Ball and Robert Ions for their kind words and valuable technical input, as well as Mike Courtnage and mum Chris Sanderson for their motivation, help and support.

Models Cass Balch, Sean Baldock, Steve Baldock, Jeremy Corrigan, Michael Courtnage, Mark Irving, Dawn Lee, Mark Rivers and Christine Sanderson.

Text and Cover Design Sara Howell
Photography Nick Brown, Michael Courtnage
Photo Scanning GH Graphics, St Leonard's on Sea, East Sussex
Drawings Michael Courtnage
Printed and bound in Great Britain by Bell & Bain Ltd., Glasgow

Contents

Introduction

I first became interested in Soft Tissue Release when it cured my own injury.

Sport has always been the love of my life and, after taking a degree in Sports Studies and qualifying to be a massage therapist with the London School of Sports Massage (LSSM), it became my career as well as my hobby. Using the massage techniques and expertise I had been trained in, I began to have considerable success not only in preventative work but also in treating sporting injuries. My professional success flourished. My fulfilment in sport, however, plummeted when at the end of 1991, I sustained a hip injury. I was blighted with injury myself and could not run.

I tried various specialists who used differing techniques. I had a thorough biomechanical assessment that revealed no significant deficiency so I was not prescribed orthotics. A chiropractor worked on the sacroiliac joint which was stiff. One very impressive physiotherapist gave me an accurate diagnosis: 'gluteus medius compartment syndrome'. All these were accurate and valuable assessments but I still could not run. Any massage I had using deep stroking seemed to irritate the condition. Finally I visited an American massage therapist who lay me on my side, put a very strong elbow into my hip and told me to move my leg. I saw the light!

My professional and sporting life turned a new corner together. Soft Tissue Release – the combination of movement and manipulation – put my sporting life back on the road to recovery and sent my professional life along a new path.

Detailed, accurate and technical work to the soft tissues is often the missing link within physical therapies. A deep massage is not the answer to everything but it is a vital therapy to accompany the others. Many injuries are due to minor soft tissue dysfunction and muscle imbalance and can be solved with the right massage.

It is almost a natural development for the experienced massage therapist to start involving movement as he finds 'stubborn' areas, so there are probably numerous ways of working in a similar fashion. In this book I outline the techniques I have been finding successful over the past seven years of my experience. STR is not intended to exclude traditional massage techniques. Experience in massage therapy is the foundation for good practice in STR: involving movement and the active co-operation of the subject is a positive step forward for the skilled therapist.

My initial introduction to STR was through the London School of Sports Massage (LSSM). My knowledge has grown and evolved in this area of expertise through my own experience and liaison with other therapists. The book is not injury diagnostic but purely an insight into an efficient method for assessing and treating the soft tissues.

Part I

Introduction to Soft Tissue Release

SOFT TISSUE DYSFUNCTION

The Soft Tissues

The musculoskeletal system consists of the soft tissues: muscle, fascia, tendon and ligament, which attach across joints to the skeleton. Muscles contract and relax to maintain posture and to provide movement. They are attached to bone by tendons or an aponeurosis, which are thickened extensions of the muscle's fascia. Fascia is all encompassing and packages, supports and envelops all the body's muscles and organs. It separates different muscles yet allows them to glide smoothly beside each other. The fascial planes provide pathways for nerves, blood vessels and lymphatic vessels. Fascia, therefore, plays a key role in maintaining the 'health' of muscle. If the fascia has been torn or over-stressed its subsequent loss of elasticity will cause and maintain chronic tissue congestion.

Over-use Injury

Micro strains to muscles always occur. If an individual performs a variety of different movements in everyday life, if he has a good neutral posture, if he rests sufficiently and eats well, these strains heal and cause no problems.

This is usually not the case as many people are involved with repetitive activities, either from an occupational or from a sporting point of view, which continue to stress the affected area. Secondary tension arises around these tiny tears to protect them from further use. Repair takes place with the formation of collagenous tissue. This micro damage, secondary tension and repair can go unnoticed by the individual. However, as the activity persists over weeks, months or years, the same tissues are constantly traumatised, so the tension and fibrous tissue are maintained. The body adapts to the hypertonicity and its posture becomes altered. As fascia supports the movements of the muscle it also can shorten and become thickened.

Weaknesses, imbalance and reduced function become evident but warning signs of potential malfunction are often not heeded and possibly not even detected until the continual overload causes a breakdown. The 'breakdown' can take several forms, for example severe soft tissue trauma, a variety of tendon injury, or an annular disc tear. This is how an over-use injury is sustained. It can be accentuated by bad bio-mechanics such as poor working posture, participating in sports with faulty or incorrect equipment, performing with bad technique, building up training too quickly or sudden adaptations to training or a technique.

The following is an example of how an over-use injury can develop: a distance runner due to an increase in mileage acquires micro tears in the gluteal muscles. He slightly favours one leg during running and a subtle imbalance forms so that the gluteus maximus and medius develop more tension. The iliotibial band (ITB) shortens slightly and the tensor fasciae latae (TFL) becomes tightened. He may also develop some shortening in the lower back. All this has gone undetected by the athlete and he continues training. Before long, however he develops a sharp pain towards the lateral knee and cannot run. The ITB is grating on the lateral condyle of the femur. He perceives the injury as being in the knee and recent, but it originated much earlier in the gluteal muscles.

Injury rarely occurs in isolation and the whole pattern needs to be assessed and treated. In the above example this means the gluteal muscles, the TFL, the band itself and adherence it may have to the lateral thigh muscles. The back and deep hip flexors may need assessment and there is also likely to be associated joint reactions. A knowledge of fascial continuities will also enhance treatment and help the therapist to understand patterns of 'release' (Myers, 1997).

Fascia

An understanding of the structure of connective tissue will help explain why soft tissue techniques, such as STR, have such a powerful and positive effect in healing and maintaining the health of the musculoskeletal system.

Fascia is an all-encompassing array of different layers of fibrous connective tissue, packaging and surrounding all of the body's structures. It stems from two levels: the superficial or subcutaneous layer which wraps the whole body from head to toe, and the deep fascia which envelops the organs, viscera and muscle. Myofascia refers to fascia associated with the skeletal muscle.

All connective tissue is composed of a strong, pliable extra-cellular matrix of collagen, elastin and reticular fibres surrounded by a ground substance of water and glycosaminoglycans (GAGs). The long white fibres of collagen are the chief component of connective tissue and their tough strands give the tissue its shape, strength, resiliency and structural integrity (Juhan, 1998). The matrix is embedded with cells, such as fibroblasts and chondrocytes that rebuild the tissue when damaged (Lederman, 1997). The functions of particular connective tissues are determined by the structure of its extra-cellular matrix and ground substance. In fibrous connective tissue, such as tendons, ligaments and fascia, the ground substance contains little fluid and many fibres of collagen and elastin, forming a tough, stringy material (Juhan, 1987). Tendons have collagen fibres arranged in parallel formation for strength and rigidity whereas in ligaments they are arranged more loosely and in different directions to cope with multidirectional forces (Lederman, 1997).

The ground substance lubricates the fibres and allows them to glide over one another (Williams, 1995) and provides a medium for exchange of elements such as oxygen, nutrients and cellular waste (Juhan, 1987). The ground substance, therefore, will affect the health of the cells.

The texture of the ground substance can change from a gelatinous gel-like substance that limits movement, to a more flexible state that facilitates it. This property is known as thixotropy. Movement, soft tissue manipulation, heat and vibration maintain a porous, hydrated ground substance which allows for gaseous and nutritional exchange and the smooth gliding of collagen and elastin fibres.

Injury, chronic stress and immobility cause the ground substance to dehydrate and harden, and lead to the formation of adhesion and scar tissue. Fibroblasts migrate to the site of injury and secrete collagen. As the tissue continues to be stressed over a period of time, the collagen thickens and spreads through the fascial web. The random laying down of collagen fibres reduces the lengthening potential and thus limits the movement of connective tissue (Juhan, 1987).

As all of the skeletal muscles are supported in myofascial tissue, local injury or stress can lead to body-wide compensatory shifts. The widespread rigidity of fascial tissue locks the soft tissues into positions of strain and dysfunction and pathophysiological changes unfold. Fascial disruption can cause minuscule shifting of bones that may irritate joint surfaces and reflexively produce further soft tissue dysfunction (Chaitow, 1996). Reduced or altered movement patterns manifest, and compression of nervous tissue, blood and lymphatic vessels are compounded. The restoration of myofascial tissue is fundamental in not only releasing muscle tension but also in restoring postural misalignment, reducing neuro excitability and improving venous and lymphatic flow.

Acute and Sub-acute Injury

Major injury can be the result of a direct trauma from an external force or as a consequence to repeated micro tears (over-use). The severity of injury is judged by the amount of fibres damaged. Tearing of fibres can occur within a muscle or muscles and in more severe strains the fascia surrounding the muscle can be torn. Following any initial injury, RICE (Rest, Ice, Compression and Elevation) is the recommended first aid. Rest is vital to prevent further damage but controlled movement that does not stress the injured area in the sub-acute phase will encourage collagen fibres to align along the lines of structural stress (Lederman, 1997). Ice is analgesic and also decreases metabolic activity and reduces blood and lymph flow where bleeding and swelling are occurring. Compression should be administered carefully so as to reduce the development of swelling without curtailing circulation. Elevation is beneficial where appropriate, to help venous and lymphatic flow against gravity and also to minimise swelling.

Ligament Injury

Ligamentous tearing is generally referred to as a 'sprain'. In this book, ligaments and joint capsule membranes are generally not included in the treatment of the 'soft tissues', although they are forms of connective tissue. Ligaments can, however, be treated with STR and so are occasionally mentioned. Controlled exercise and movement has a positive effect on the recovery of ligaments as they have a relatively poor blood supply compared to muscles and tendons so healing is often slow. By administering appropriate STR the collagen turnover is increased and by ensuring that the muscles, tendons and fascia around the injury are in good condition, their repair will be enhanced.

Tendon Injury

Tendons are mechanically strong as they transfer the force of the contracting muscle to the bone; because of this, however, they lack elasticity. With any tendon injury it is necessary to treat the muscle from which it originates as well as neighbouring or other relevant soft tissues in the 'pattern' of release. Areas of congestion commonly prevail at the musculotendinous junction. Particularly where there is inflammation, treatment on the actual tendon should be limited. The following are common tendon conditions:

Tendinitis: Inflammation and scarring of the tendon itself.

Tenovaginitis: The synovial sheath around the tendon is inflamed and thickened.

Tenosynovitis: Inflammation between the synovial sheath and the tendon.

Peritendinitis: Inflammation and thickening of the paratenon. (A paratenon being the membranous tissue around tendons that have no synovial sheath, e.g. Achilles tendon).

MASSAGE AND STR

Massage Techniques

As well as having its own specific attributes, STR has all the physiological benefits of traditional massage. Massage can increase venous and lymphatic drainage. The increase in interstitial pressure during and after massage allows for easier fluid absorption so that fresh blood can enter fatigued or traumatised areas. Adhesive tissues can be mobilised and scar tissue broken into smaller particles for phagocytosis and lymphatic absorption to occur.

Massage strokes can stretch muscle fibres longitudinally and improve collagen flexibility.

There are advanced soft tissue techniques which bring into play the nervous system to over-ride reflex holding patterns. Performed correctly, neuromuscular techniques (NMT) will eradicate tension areas and scar tissue. STR can sometimes involve this neuromuscular element, as the treatment on occasion is painful.

Methods that specifically target the connective tissues are also highly effective. By addressing the connective tissues with a 'CTM' lock (*see* page 27) STR can incorporate the effectiveness of Connective Tissue Massage (CTM).

STR and Research

All tissue has conductive ability. When myofascial disruption occurs, a reduction in the electric potential is generated. Research suggests that dense collagen reduces or impedes electrical flow through the tissue, thus reducing the activity of the local fascial cells. The thixotropic quality of myofascia means that when it shortens or thickens it 'dries out' and the ground substance turns from a watery solution which facilitates movement, to a less flexible gel which limits movement.

Application of pressure brings about a solution and rehydration. Removal of the pressure causes a re-gelling but the tissues will have improved in both conductive ability and water content (J. L. Oschman, 1997). This boosts electrical activity and improves the neuromuscular relationship.

Movement is essential in the repair and maintenance of healthy tissue. It provides direction for deposition of collagen and encourages vascular regeneration. Movement also lubricates and hydrates connective tissue by improving the balance in the ground substance between the GAG's and the water. This will reduce the potential for adhesion formation (Lederman, 1997).

Research with tissue cultures highlight the importance of both stress and motion to healing. Lederman, 1997, also states that 'active techniques will stimulate muscle fibre regeneration, a normal ratio of muscle to connective tissue elements and the development of neuromuscular connections.' Combination treatment of pressure and movement, therefore, should have a significant positive effect on the quality of the myofascial tissue. When working on passive tissues, they present as relatively soft and pressure is diffused by their softness; deep connective tissue restrictions may not get enough mechanical energy to cause thixotropic change (Juhan, 1987). If pressure and movement are applied together with muscular contraction, tissue density is significantly increased. This increases the pressure delivery through the myofascial tissue and will enhance the effectiveness of treatment (Lowe, 1999).

Combining concentric muscle contraction with a specific 'broadening' pressure into the myofascial tissue facilitates a greater mobilisation of the connective tissues (Lowe, 1999). Longitudinal stress may also positively influence the pattern of myofascial tissue (Cantu and Grodin, 1992) and the application of longitudinal strokes while the tissue undergoes eccentric contraction effectively stretches and lengthens the connective tissues.

It would seem that treatment could be more rapid and the pressures applied by the therapist reduced when pressure and external movement of the tissues are combined.

The only currently available research into the technique of Soft Tissue Release (STR) is a preliminary single case study on a hemiplegic stroke patient. Barnard, 2000, found that the application of STR to the muscles controlling elbow flexion and supination, increased elbow Range of Movement (ROM) and reduced elbow flexor spasticity. The study also showed the positive effects to have lasted.

There is huge scope for research into STR as there is a lack of empirical evidence to show that the technique is effective. Palpation skills are difficult to measure and so, as is often the case, research is lagging behind clinical experience.

Prevention of Injury

Regular stretching and massage are essential in maintaining condition of muscles and reducing the possibility of injury. If areas of soft tissue malfunction are detected, they can be dispersed prior to a more major injury forming. Strong individual muscles will resist stress better than muscles that are shortened and adhered. In competitive sport for example, where intense training is necessary for success, muscles are continually being shortened, micro-torn and fatigued. Massage will elongate and nourish the shortened tissue, enabling it to repair and adapt to the demands of training. Treatment will vary according to severity and amount of training but in most cases potential problem areas can be detected prior to dysfunction or reduced performance.

Over-use Injury

When dealing with injuries caused by over-use, massage comes into its own. With STR large areas can be assessed fairly quickly so severe problems of hypertonicity and muscle shortening can be detected and addressed, prior to focusing on a specific spot. Correct usage of STR can separate and re-align adhesions, break down collagen tissue and lengthen chronically shortened fibres. STR can stretch fascia specifically to reduce pressure on a muscle. All this enables muscles to become nourished, pliable and flexible so that they may contract and relax without resistance. So, whether breakdown is a result of sporting activities such as long distance running, or from repetitive everyday pursuits which stress the musculature, such as sustained postures, a course of treatments enables re-balancing and a return to full function to occur. Where chronic inflammation is present, ice can be used alongside treatment.

Traumatic Injury

Correct treatment, even in relatively minor injuries or low-grade strains, is essential to ensure that full mobility and strength is regained. Massage techniques in conjunction with RICE will help the healing processes. Massage away from the site of injury during inflammatory stages is beneficial because it maintains good circulation, thereby encouraging drainage of any swelling. For example in an ankle inversion sprain the calf muscles may be treated. In the sub-acute and repair phase of healing, careful use of STR can be done to encourage collagen to align in an orderly fashion. In the case of the ankle this may be treatment to the peroneal muscles and their tendons and the lateral ligament complex as well as maintaining balance by treating all tendons which cross the ankle. STR, being a functional treatment modality, is an ideal technique given the necessity for rehabilitation to consist of 'active rest'. As recovery continues, compensatory problems may develop. In an ankle sprain, plantar muscles of the foot may tighten due to subtly altered bio-mechanics and tensions can form in the other leg where limping has occurred. These problems can be minimised with massage, efficient checks and STR.

STR in Conjunction With Other Therapies

Most injuries contain components of soft tissue damage, which can cause localised pain and dysfunction, so careful administering of appropriate massage will contribute to healing even if other forms of therapy are also required. For instance, if there is a mechanical misalignment or restriction, mobilisations may be essential for normal function to resume and, in the case of adverse neurological tension, gliding the nerve at the tissue interface may be necessary. In both of these situations practitioners trained in these skills are needed for accurate diagnosis and management of the injury. Skilled use of STR, however, will aid both these forms of treatment. If the soft tissues are free to move in a controlled and separate way, they will facilitate joint manipulation or nerve mobilisation and help maintain the effects of the other treatment.

After periods of immobilisation, such as when a plaster of paris has been removed from a limb following a fracture, STR can be used effectively to reduce scarring and oedema and return flexibility with elasticity to the soft tissues. This enables strength, proprioceptive and co-ordination gains. The same is true of post-operative situations where incisions and periods of rest severely affect the condition of the soft tissues. Any incision will cause scarring and prolonged rest results in loss of strength and reduced function; STR can help with the rehabilitation.

Important Considerations

Massage, including STR, is a safe therapy, providing that contra-indications are understood. There are occasions where massage is detrimental or dangerous so an understanding of contra-indications prior to any massage is imperative. Massage can have amazing results in preventative care and is highly effective in treating minor soft tissue injuries or over-use conditions; but it is necessary to liaise with or to seek a diagnosis from a qualified medical practitioner prior to treating complex injuries solely with massage. Massage therapists need to recognise their strengths and limitations. Diagnosis from the medical health care practitioner, prior to massage, allows an integrative approach that allows practitioners to ensure that the STR treatment suits the subject's needs.

As with all massage, it is important to avoid over-treating areas with STR. When working on particularly congested tissues there may be some discomfort during release. Treat systematically and holistically rather than repeatedly going over the same area or location of dysfunction. This will minimise any bruising due to tissue damage during the massage.

ASSESSING THE SOFT TISSUES

Texture

Experience gives the massage therapist the ability to distinguish between the various kinds of soft tissue according to how they feel. When relaxed and in good condition, muscle should feel soft and pliable. Tendons, being fibrous extensions of the muscles' fascia, feel firmer and more 'stringy'. Where there is specialised thickening of fascia, such as the iliotibial band and the thoracolumbar fascia, tissue will also feel firmer and less resilient.

An overall assessment of relevant tissues is necessary to evaluate their condition. Many deep muscles are not directly palpable. 'Release' of superficial muscles so that they are supple and relaxed, enables the therapist to work into and affect the deep muscles. In some instances only the border of a muscle may be reached. This is the case with the quadratus lumborum where pressure is attained laterally and directed towards the vertebrae. The stretch is produced so that the fascia and outer muscle fibres are released thereby nourishing and freeing the muscle as a whole.

General variations will occur due to age, sex, fitness, type of sport or activity the body undergoes, lack of activity, level of activity or competition, occupation and previous injury. However, poor texture may be identified and categorised under the following headings:

1. Hypertonicity and Muscle Tightness

Tightness in a muscle represents both increase in tone and decrease in the resting length of the muscle. When a muscle is hypertonic it has too much muscle tone, but it may either have decreased or increased resting muscle length. On palpation, the fibres feel resistant and lack pliability.

2. Adhesions

Following inflammation and the formation of fibrous tissue, adhesion of fascia can occur; this usually occurs as longitudinal bands of adherence. They feel woody and stringy and may 'flick' if being palpated transversely. In the text, 'separation' of neighbouring muscle groups is frequently mentioned and refers to the separating of adherence that may be occurring between the muscles.

3. Scar Tissue

Inflammation and repair can result in the formation of a collagenous scar. Scar tissue is new collagen that has been secreted by fibroblasts. It lacks mobility, extensibility and strength and can feel gritty, like marbles, or, in severe cases, hard and solid.

4. Oedema and Swelling

Oedema and swelling are caused by an excess of tissue fluid following injury and the subsequent inflammatory response. Chronic swelling can occur where tightness and scarring compress capillaries and lymphatics, curtailing the flow of fluid in and out of the area (ensure that oedema is not symptomatic of a more serious medical condition). The area can feel spongy and pitting of the tissue may occur.

5. General Rigidity of Superficial Fascia and Myofascia

These are large body areas which feel hard and the connective tissue feels bound down to the underlying structures. 'Skin rolling' and fascial 'lifting' are difficult to perform and can be painful for the subject. Compartment syndrome occurs where the bulk of the muscle exceeds the capacity of its encompassing myofascia. This may be because the myofascia becomes so tight and thickened that, even when the muscle is relaxed, there is an increased intramuscular pressure that causes pain. Alternatively, the fascia can be 'normal' but the muscle itself over-developed as a result of training.

Inflammation

Working directly on inflammation should be avoided because it will slow down healing. Major inflammation following an obvious trauma will present painfully, red and warm to the touch. Working *around* the inflammation will ensure that it is well nourished and, by keeping the surrounding tissues free, encourage healing and decongestion of the area.

If an area is proving sensitive, maintain a pressure for seven seconds (the seven second test). If the pain eases or stays the same, then the area can be worked on. If it worsens, there is probably inflammation so it should not be worked on directly.

Muscle Balance

Muscles can be classified into various categories depending on their role within the musculoskeletal system. Some muscles are chiefly involved with stability and posture whilst others are more directly involved with providing dynamic movement. Classification is very useful to the practitioner seeking to restore balance, but it is important to realise that it is not always clear cut. Muscle grouping is still a developing area and there are a few different classification models. Recent research has classified muscles into; local and global stabilisers and global mobilisers (Comerford, M., Mottram, M., 2000).

1. Joint
2. Muscle in balance
3. Inhibited muscle
4. Tight muscle

Figure 1: Comparative illustration of muscle in balance compared to an inhibited and tight muscle.

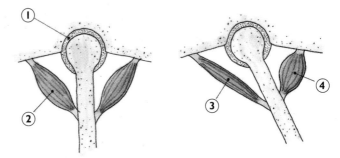

Stabilisers tend to be deep, single joint muscles that help maintain posture over sustained periods. They contract alongside other stabilisers to support and maintain position, or control movement. They are generally rich in slow twitch fibres, predominantly aerobic and slow to fatigue.

Local stabilisers are unable to provide significant joint movement. They contract isometrically to increase joint stiffness for segmental control of motion. Examples of these are the transversus abdominis, multifidis, psoas, interspinales, vastus medialis, lower fibres of the trapezius and the deep cervical flexors.

Global stabilisers function to stabilise and provide some joint movement. They control the range of movement, generally through eccentric muscle contraction and maintain posture through isometric effort. They can also contribute to movement through concentric contraction. Examples include the serratus anterior and the posterior two thirds of the gluteus medius, gluteus maximus, spinalis, longus coli and the oblique abdominals.

Mobilisers tend to be more superficial and provide larger range of movement for fast, dynamic requirements. They can perform under aerobic and anaerobic conditions and contain high levels of fast twitch muscle fibres. Examples of these are the levator scapulae, scalenes, latissimus dorsi, iliocostalis, rectus abdominis, tensor fasciae latae and the hamstrings.

Through dysfunction, local stabilisers are likely to become inhibited and slow to activate. Global stabilisers are prone to inhibition that may manifest itself as lengthening and weakening of the muscles. Stabilisers subsequently become unable to provide a stable base for other muscles to work from.

Mobilisers, on the other hand, tend to take on the failed stability role in addition to their own and over time become stressed, over active and tight. A dominant tight mobiliser pulling in one direction, with an inhibited stabiliser, unable to maintain position or control movement, against it, will cause imbalance (*see* figure 1). This will negatively affect joint alignment and movement. If maintained, postural misalignment and altered movement patterns can result in over-use injury.

Neutral joint position and posture together with controlled motion place minimal strain on the musculoskeletal system and facilitates its smooth and efficient function. To maintain these, the stabilisers must activate quickly and effectively enough and the mobilisers muscles need to be pliable, relaxed and of adequate length for their specific activity requirements.

Soft tissue techniques, such as STR, can provide fast and effective release for tight muscles. By relaxing and lengthening them, it becomes easier for the subject to engage his inhibited muscles.

One, among many examples, from my clinical experience is with patello-femoral tracking conditions. I have treated numerous athletes suffering from this, who have been prescribed strengthening exercises for the vastus medialis to no avail. 'Releasing' tightness in the vastus lateralis, however, quickly resolved their complaints. Another very common example of muscle imbalance occurs in the lower and upper fibres of the trapezius. Tight upper fibres and weak lower fibres can contribute to neck, shoulder and shoulder girdle dysfunction. Many people who have experienced poor results from performing exercises aimed at engaging the lower trapezius fibres, have subsequently responded extremely well once STR has been applied to release the upper fibres.

This is not to say that specific exercises do not a have a place, as they play an essential role in maintaining the beneficial effects of manual therapies during and following a course of treatment. Re-educational exercises will improve motor control, strengthen and reactivate inhibited muscles and stretch short and tight muscles. Exercises such as Yoga, Pilates, Feldenkrais and the Alexander Technique are excellent modalities for re-balancing the musculoskeletal system, with a strong emphasis on 'core stability' and muscle lengthening.

In conjunction with such re-educational regimes, STR can help restore muscle balance, postural misalignment and efficient movement patterns.

Part 2
STR the Technique

The technique is administered simply by applying and maintaining a pressure, or 'locking' into the relevant tissues whilst simultaneously stretching away aligning fibres.

ADMINISTERING STR

The Technique

First the fibres are located. They are then 'locked' into by applying an appropriate pressure. This pressure is maintained whilst a stretch is produced by moving a limb; the limb can be moved either by the therapist or by the active participation of the subject. This produces a powerful release where tissues are adhering. Movement and localised lengthening of the affected fibres has occurred in conjunction with separation or movement of the lesion with the 'locking in' pressure.

When conducting a general treatment, the area is initially warmed with massage strokes and the use of oil or lotion. Alternatively the muscles can be warmed-up with light passive STR using a broad locking technique. Progression to specific STR will facilitate in the detection of adhesive tissue so should be conducted even in a maintenance massage. If a problem area is uncovered, working between the muscle borders to stretch the fascia and within the muscle itself are necessary. It is not essential to cover every section of the muscle, as releasing one specific area will cause neighbouring fibres and fascia to soften and stretch. The lock should be achieved carefully and maintained whilst a stretch is initiated. If working close to bone the lock should always be angled away from the bony surface to avoid crushing of the tissue and bruising. If in doubt over the acuteness of an injury, conduct the 'seven second test' (*see* page 19).

Benefits Over Stretching Alone

If a fibrous or adhered area is present in a muscle that is predominantly strong and flexible, that muscle as a whole may be stretched without the congested area itself being stretched. The stretch alone is not enough to separate the 'gluing' of these particular muscle fibres. Muscles can be flexible without necessarily being in good condition. With STR this specific area can be targeted and locked still while its neighbouring tissues are specifically elongated, thereby focusing on the restriction.

Benefits Over Traditional Massage Strokes Alone

When administering most massage techniques, the tissues remain passive whilst the therapist glides through them or works on and across them. With STR a specific position within the tissues is acquired and it is then the tissues themselves which are moved and elongated. This makes textural assessment procedures easier. Therapists can pinpoint specific areas more quickly, particularly where there may be several muscle layers with fibres going in different directions. With the stretch, the fibres are re-arranged and elongated for efficient function. Complex soft tissue dysfunction, where many muscle groups and holding patterns are involved, can be solved because of specificity of the pressure and the stretch.

FACTORS TO CONSIDER

1. Types of STR

There are basically three types of STR: Passive, Active and Weight-bearing. All three involve movement but in active and weight-bearing STR the subject produces the movement whereas in passive STR the therapist moves the limb. Passive work provides a good release and can be very relaxing (*see* figure 2).

Active STR is more powerful and should be preceded by passive work or other massage to warm-up the area. Progression to active work is more energy efficient for the therapist, allowing concentration to centre on the application of the pressure. Many subjects prefer to become actively involved with, or to control a particular release, especially when areas are painful to work with (*see* figure 3).

Applying resistance during active STR may enhance the 'release' in some cases. As the subject attempts to produce a stretch, but is resisted from doing so, isometric muscle contraction takes place in the antagonist muscles, and because of this there is an enhanced relaxation in the muscle undergoing treatment. This effect is known as 'reciprocal inhibition' (RI) (*see* figure 4).

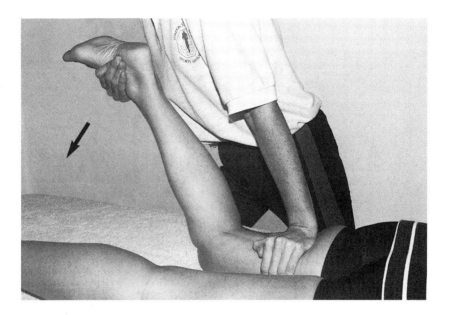

Figure 2: Passive STR.

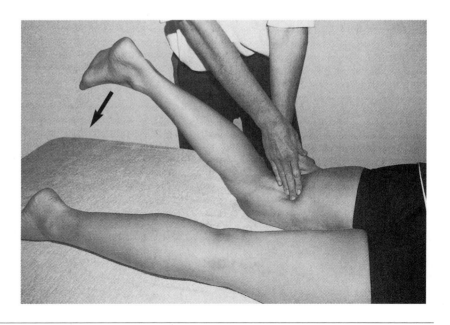

Figure 3: Active STR.

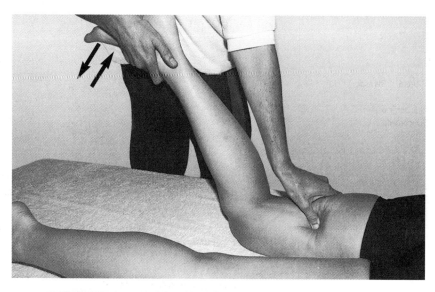

Figure 4: Resisted STR.

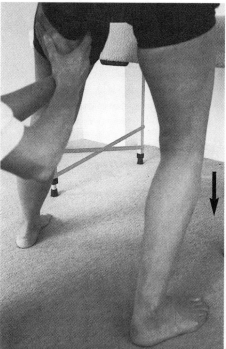

Figure 5: Weight-bearing STR.

Weight-bearing STR is highly effective in returning an area to full function. The muscles are under tension and a degree of eccentric contraction may be occurring to control the required movement. Manipulation under this tension may be very severe, so should be the last stage in any treatment programme (*see* figure 5).

2. Application of Pressure or 'Lock'

How the pressure, or lock, is applied and the direction and angle of pressure is important for effective results. The lock can be used to lengthen or traverse the target fibres. It can also be used to delve between muscle groups, to isolate tendons ((*see* figure 7) or to separate bellies within a muscle (*see* figure 8). A form of friction is being created where pressure is attained, and the movement is made by the subject either passively or actively. Friction breaks the fibrous tissue binding the fibres and the movement enables this to happen in the correct direction to re-align them.

Specific Attention to the Fascia

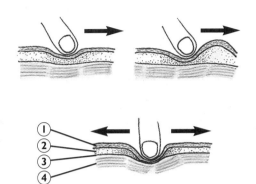

Figure 6: CTM lock.

(i) Superficial fascia
(subcutaneous layer)

(ii) Myofascia

1. Skin
2. Subcutaneous layer
3. Myofascia
4. Muscle

A connective tissue massage (CTM) lock is designed to work specifically on fascia. Depth should be attained before slowly gliding the fascia; once there is resistance, the lock should be moved 2–3cms further. Once this is achieved, it is maintained whilst the movement occurs (*see* figure 6).

3. Maintenance of Pressure

Pressure is maintained during the stretch, whatever the type of lock. The release occurs with the movement from the subject. The lock is maintained, while the fibres around are moving; this may cause the lock to jump or flicker but the movement is still being produced functionally by the subject not by moving the lock.

4. The Stretch

Maximal stretching is not the best way to release specific problem areas; the stretch should be localised. The basic principle behind STR is that congested fibres can be targeted more accurately. In some instances the stretch may involve only the tiniest of movements. Also, on occasions it is necessary to shorten a muscle prior to locking in, to relax the fibres so that an effective lock can be applied.

There may be many different ways to produce a stretch, particularly where muscles have more than one action. In some cases the therapist may even choose to combine movements; for example, when treating the biceps brachii, the elbow can be extended and pronated as the pressure is applied. Where a more severe stretch is being attained the therapist should guide the subject into one movement and follow it with a further stretch. For example, in the hamstrings the hip may be flexed first as the pressure is applied and then a further stretch reached as the knee is extended.

5. Flexibility

STR is a very useful technique for subjects who require flexibility for whatever reason. It may be that the muscle or tendon fibres are shortened because of over-use or imbalance, or it may be that the nature of the relevant activity necessitates a high level of flexibility such as in gymnastics or martial arts. In these cases full stretching should be incorporated within STR only after the tissues have been worked on thoroughly. It is also important to note that range of movement must be tested prior to instructing a subject to move into an extreme stretch.

6. In Conjunction with Muscle Energy Techniques

Muscle Energy Techniques (MET) can be used to great effect alongside STR. MET refers to stretching techniques which involve the subject's own muscular energy to help release holding tension. For example, following an isometric muscle contraction there is a period of relaxation called 'post isometric relaxation' (PIR). A therapist experienced in this can use this principle to enhance muscle relaxation and, therefore, its stretching capability. The use of the principle of 'reciprocal inhibition' (RI) has already been mentioned with reference to 'resisted STR'.

7. Discomfort during Application

Where tissues are so severely adhered and fibrous that it may be painful to separate them, STR has two advantages over other techniques. Firstly, there is a pleasant, momentary relief when the pressure is released, even if a new lock is being sought. Secondly, the subject feels in control of his own discomfort. This may be particularly the case with high performance sports people who willingly put themselves through painful training sessions for success in their event!

AIDS TO APPLICATION OF STR

Tools

As with all massage, the tools of the trade are; fingers, thumbs, knuckles, whole hands, forearms and elbows. A good working posture should be adopted so that deep pressure can be applied when necessary with minimal strain to the therapist. The larger superficial muscles with general shortening are treated first with broader pressure points such as the

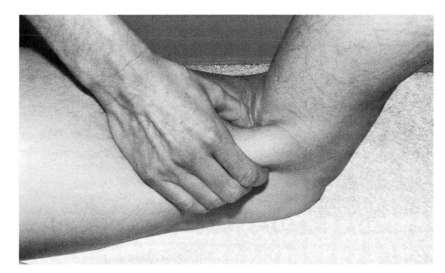

Figure 7: The tendon is being isolated for a specific release.

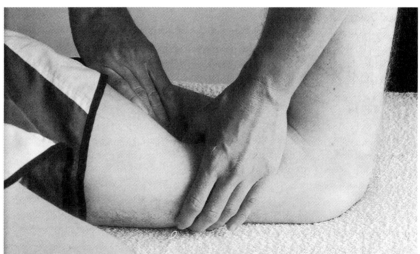

Figure 8: Separation of muscle bellies.

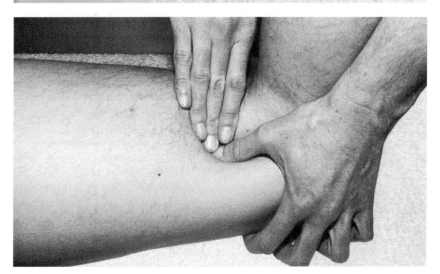

Figure 9: The thumb is being reinforced by the fingers on the other hand.

forearm or heel of the hand. Prior to working the deeper muscles, the area is assessed and released of tension so that the superficial muscles can be reached through with minimal discomfort. Deep work can be done with a smaller surface area such as the thumb or knuckle, so that the force applied is greater. Specific deep pressure often requires reinforcement such as the weight of the opposing hand, and body weight behind it, to protect the therapist from joint damage or fatigue (*see* figure 9). For experienced practitioners, wooden pegs are available which fit in the hand and assist in the achievement of deep pressures. These have to be used sparingly and with intelligence, as the therapist will have lost the sensitivity he would normally have when using his own hands or elbows.

Ideally a correctly positioned treatment couch is required for the delivery of good massage, but STR is a highly adaptive technique which will test the ingenuity of the therapist. Treatment can be conducted through clothes, at sporting events where there are no facilities, where events are cold and exposed and where time is a limiting factor.

Tips to Ensure Effective Administering of STR

- Lock slowly and precisely. Avoid 'poking' or 'shoving' the tissue.
- Gradually apply the 'lock' to the congested or 'stuck' layer at a transverse or oblique angle.
- Follow your subject's breathing. Gain your depth as he exhales to maintain his relaxation. When working very deep or in severely congested areas it may take two or three exhalations to reach the 'lock' you require.
- Passively guiding your subject through the stretch prior to him performing it will ensure that he completes the movement correctly.
- Asking your subject for the movement will engage the adhering tissue. Telling him when to breathe will increase his awareness and help him to relax. This will also allow him to feel that he is playing an important role in the session.
- Analyse where to go next and move on slowly.
- Avoid spending too long in any one place if nothing seems to be happening – move on.
- Release occurs in many different ways not just where you are focusing. Allow your awareness to move beyond the tissue you are working on.
- Stay in verbal contact with your subject asking questions like, 'Are you okay?', 'How does that feel?'

Part 3
Lower Limb

THE PELVIC GIRDLE

The pelvic girdle is strong and stable with minimal mobility; it joins the lower limb to the spine transferring the weight of the body to the legs. The maintenance of good pelvic posture during sitting, standing or moving is critical in ensuring the efficient functioning of the area. Balance and strength in the trunk and hip muscles are the key to achieving this.

The lumbosacral junction articulates the sacrum and the lumbar vertebrae and is vulnerable to injury. The iliolumbar ligament is a particularly strong ligament that helps to stabilise the joint. It is a specialised extension of the thoracolumbar fascia (anterior and middle sections) originating from L5 and joining to the posterior inner lip of the iliac crest. It is imperative to address the connective tissues around this area as constant stress particularly from sitting, standing and bending, will cause fascial thickening and rigidity leading to pain and dysfunction.

The sacroiliac joint connects the sacrum to the pelvic girdle and transfers body weight from the trunk to the leg, so it is important to consider it in any treatment of the area. Anteriorly the pelvis joins at the symphysis pubis. Tendinous fibres of the rectus abdominis, external oblique and the adductor longus overlay the cartilaginous disc. This offers the joint extra strength and stability. When presented with osteoitis pubis, these are the muscles that should be treated.

THE HIPS

The enormous strength and musculature of the hip joint is necessary to cater for dynamic and controlled propulsion. The hips support the weight of the body and also transfer the weight powerfully, to the opposing leg, in a range of different weight-bearing activities from walking to running and jumping. Full range of movement and strength in the hips will encourage a bio-mechanically efficient and smooth gait.

Hip Extension

Major Muscles: Gluteus maximus. *Hamstrings*: semimembranosus, semitendinosus and biceps femoris (long head). Adductor magnus (vertical fibres).

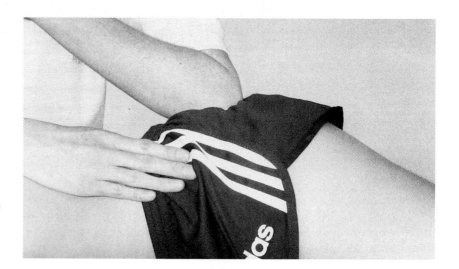

Figure 10: Deep pressure in the gluteus maximus as the hip is flexed.

Gluteus Maximus

The gluteus maximus is a very strong muscle involved with powerful hip extension particularly from a flexed starting position. Movements such as stair climbing, rising from a seated position or squat, walking uphill and running, especially fast running which requires great drive and power, employ this muscle. As the gluteus maximus arises from the lower fascia of the back, it is consequently involved with trunk extension from a flexed position. It is also an important lateral rotator so will affect foot plant. Static build-up of tensions can also occur in the gluteus maximus because of its contribution to supporting the body's weight in the seated position; contraction will take the body's weight off the ischial tuberosities. Strains to this muscle are more likely to occur at its origins along the sacrum and iliac crest.

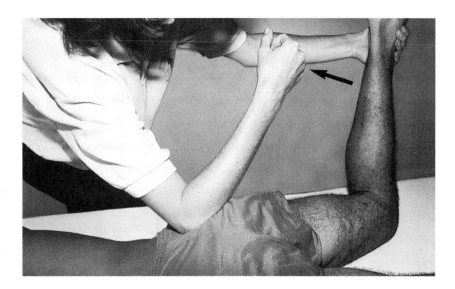

Figure 11: Deep pressure in the gluteus maximus as the hip is medially rotated.

Lateral Rotation

Major Muscles: Gluteus maximus, posterior fibres of the gluteus medius, sartorius. Deep lateral rotators: piriformis, obturator internus, obturator externus, gemellus superior, gemellus inferior, quadratus femoris and psoas major.

These muscles are important in stabilising all hip movements by preventing excessive medial rotation. The piriformis is often problematic. It is involved in the seated position as an abductor. It is also an important stabiliser. The sciatic nerve runs beneath this muscle and in 25% of the population may actually run through the muscle. It can become adhered to the piriformis and give sciatic symptoms (posterior thigh). Sciatica resulting from this is known as piriformis syndrome and responds very well to STR.

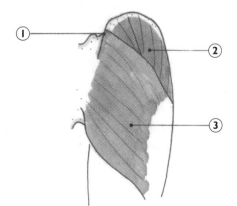

1. *Posterior superior iliac spine (PSIS)*
2. *Gluteus medius*
3. *Gluteus maximus*

Figure 12: Superficial hip muscles.

Medial Rotation

Major Muscles: Anterior fibres of the gluteus medius, gluteus minimus and TFL, pectineus, adductor longus, adductor brevis, adductor magnus.

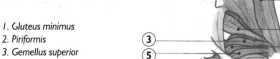

1. Gluteus minimus
2. Piriformis
3. Gemellus superior
4. Obturator internus
5. Gemellus inferior
6. Quadratus femoris

Figure 13: Deep hip muscles.

Gluteus Maximus and the Deep Lateral Rotators – Treatment

In prone position, apply pressure at points off the gluteal attachments by locking in and moving away from the iliac crest and away from the sacrum, while the subject attempts to flex his hip by pushing his knee into the table. Given that the lock is precise, a small stretch will be felt. To obtain a more significant stretch in the muscle as a whole, treat the muscle in a side lying position where full flexion can be obtained with the subject actively drawing his knee in (*see* figure 10). So that this movement can be controlled, the subject can hold his own knee and flex the hip once the lock is secured.

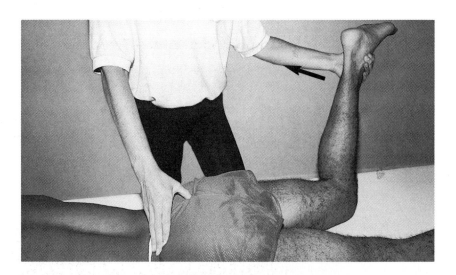

Figure 14: A pressure in the gluteus maximus with the thumb while the hip is rotated. This can be done actively to allow for thumb reinforcement.

Alternatively, with the subject in prone position, and the knee flexed to 90 degrees, gently rotate the leg medially and laterally. This will in itself indicate major tension. Lock in appropriately, broad surface first, away from the sacrum, then away from the iliac crest, each time applying the pressure, then medially rotating the leg and releasing the pressure to return the leg to the starting point (*see* figures 11 and 14). Systematically cover the whole of the gluteus maximus area and once it is relaxed and stretched, progress to the deep rotators. Angle your elbow gently through towards the piriformis which can be located halfway between the sacrum and the greater trochanter. Ensure that the relaxation of the muscles is maintained.

The other rotators can also be affected, although they are difficult to differentiate. The quadratus femoris can be reached by gliding away from the ischial tuberosity and under the gluteus maximus. Once any one of these deep pressures is attained, hold the pressure and medially rotate slowly, then promptly release the pressure.

Medial Rotators – Treatment

The gluteus medius and minimus can be treated as one, the minimus lying directly under the medius. Apply pressure in the gluteus medius, away from the iliac crest and laterally rotate the leg. Another useful manoeuvre is with the subject supine. Link into the medius with the fingers of one hand reinforced with the other hand and slowly pull the fibres transversely very slightly. Lock his opposing hip with your knee to stabilise the pelvis while he actively rotates his leg, medially if the posterior fibres are locked and laterally if the anterior fibres are locked. It is also possible to work the TFL well here with the same method.

Sacroiliac Joint Area – Treatment

Once the hips and lower back have been warmed-up, treatment of this area can occur. Position the subject on his side and apply a CTM lock away from the posterior superior iliac spine (PSIS) and instruct him into minimal hip flexion (*see* figure 15). Progress to the 'V', between the PSIS and the lumbosacral joint, and apply a CTM lock, again guiding the subject into hip flexion (*see* also page 66).

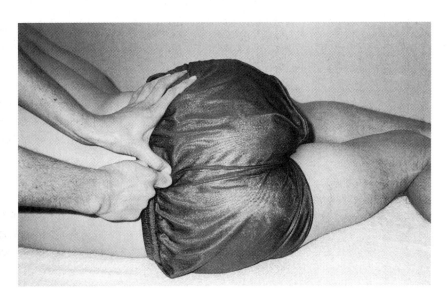

Figure 15: A CTM lock away from the PSIS as the subject flexes the hip.

Hamstrings

Muscles: Semimembranosus, semitendinosus and biceps femoris.

The hamstrings work with the gluteus maximus to extend the hip if the knee is mostly or completely extended. They also assist the gluteus maximus in extending the spine from a flexed position. If hip extension is not occurring then the hamstrings are also powerful knee flexors. When the knee is semi-flexed some rotation can also occur.

Hamstring strains are common in sports involving sprinting where the muscles are used powerfully. Sprinters in athletics are renowned for problems here. The sprint starting position puts huge stress on the three hamstrings which are working around two strong movements: the trunk is rising from crouched position, while the hip extends powerfully to drive the body forward. A good sprinter may not be running fully erect until 25 metres into his sprint. Strains occur towards the origin or in the belly of the muscle more commonly than at the insertion points.

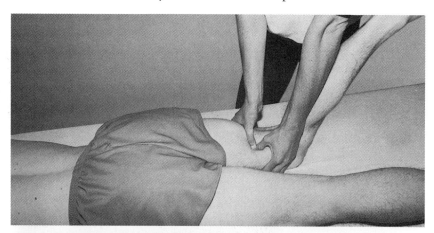

Figure 16: Pressure in the hamstrings as the knee is extended.

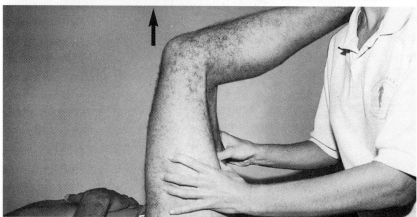

Figure 17: STR in the hamstrings facilitating a greater stretch.

Hamstrings – Treatment

There are many different ways of treating the hamstrings and it is important to adapt depending on the size and condition of the muscles. As a whole, they are best treated initially from a prone position for initial investigation (*see* figure 16). With the knee flexed to 90 degrees, apply locks towards the origin as the knee is straightened each time. Treat from the tendons of insertion to the origins locating the three hamstrings. Delve between the muscle groups separating adherence. In a supine position a greater stretch can be achieved. Support his lower leg on your shoulder whilst locking with the thumbs, then instruct him to extend his knee. Variations using knuckles or elbows may prove easier to administer (*see* figures 17, 18 and 19).

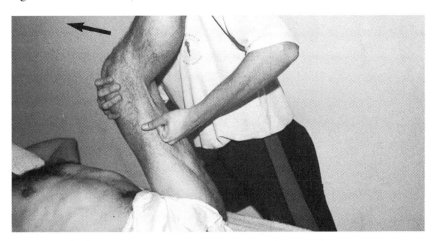

Figure 18: Use of knuckles for a deeper but less precise 'lock'.

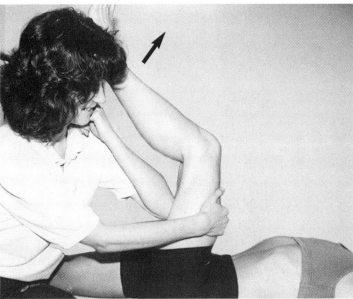

Figure 19: Use of the elbow for a deep pressure in the hamstrings.

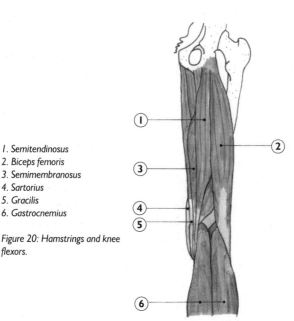

1. Semitendinosus
2. Biceps femoris
3. Semimembranosus
4. Sartorius
5. Gracilis
6. Gastrocnemius

Figure 20: Hamstrings and knee flexors.

With the subject supine, STR may be administered on and away from the origin with him flexing his hip while the lock is directed towards the insertions. He may need to hold the leg just above and behind the knee and pull it up into flexion for the best control (see figure 21). The pressure should be attained slowly because any adhesion will be very sensitive. It is also possible to work this area with the subject in side lying position ensuring that his leg is supported while he flexes his hip.

Weight-bearing STR in the hamstrings may provide powerful results. With the subject standing, apply a pressure as he slowly stretches (see figure 22).

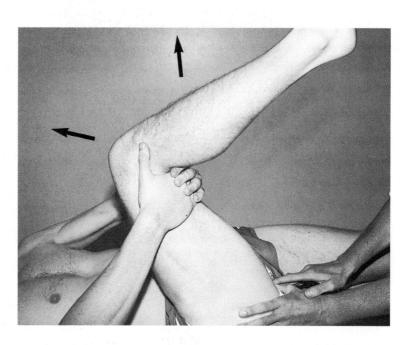

Figure 21: Pressure away from the hamstring origin as the hip is flexed or the knee extended.

Hip Flexion

Major Muscles: Rectus femoris, sartorius, TFL, pectineus, iliacus, psoas major and psoas minor (not always present).

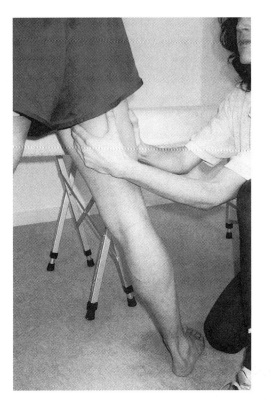

Figure 22: STR on the hamstrings close to the origin in a weight-bearing position.

All of the hip flexors position the pelvis forwards; if they become adhered or tight they become less effective in holding the pelvis up in a neutral position. This can be associated with weak abdominal muscles and subsequent lordosis. If this is the case, specific isolated abdominal strengthening is vital and STR to the hip flexors will facilitate the strength gains. The psoas is strong and powerful, and is a major postural muscle. When the insertions are fixed, the psoas assists in flexing the trunk from a lying position. During treatment, both sides should always be considered when presented with any lumbago conditions, lordosis, or other postural deficiencies. The iliacus and psoas are often termed as the 'iliopsoas'.

Hip Flexors – Treatment

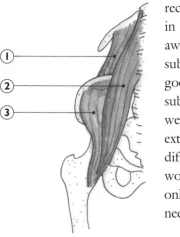

1. Quadratus lumborum
2. Psoas
3. Iliacus

Figure 23: Deep hip flexors and quadratus lumborum.

With the client supine on the table, treat the rectus femoris, sartorius and TFL by locking in gently but firmly (this can be ticklish) away from the origin, then instruct the subject to tilt the pelvis (posterior tilt). A good alternative is to work these with the subject in side lying position. Support his leg well, lock appropriately and take the leg into extension (*see* figure 24). This can be difficult with the heavier leg, but with active work, a good lock can be maintained and only a tiny amount of hip extension is needed for an effective release (*see* figure 25).

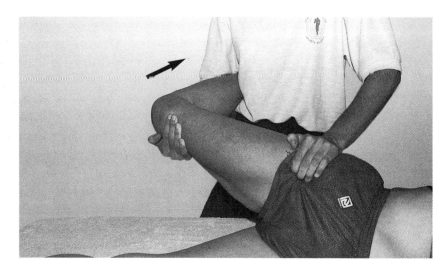

Figure 24: Pressure in the rectus femoris as the therapist provides hip extension.

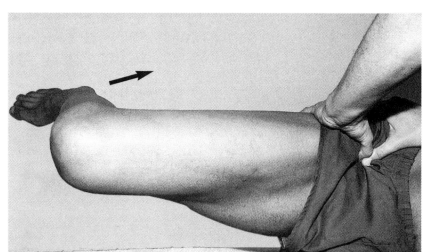

Figure 25: Pressure in the rectus femoris as the subject moves into hip extension.

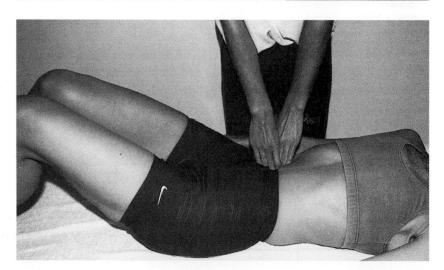

Figure 26: Pressure is attained slowly towards the psoas muscle prior to the subject extending the hip to the table.

With the iliopsoas, extreme care and subject relaxation are essential for good results. Position the subject supine with knees bent; position your fingers halfway between the last rib and the linea alba; as he exhales, gently drop towards the muscle then stop as he inhales and wait to go deeper for his second and maybe even third exhalation (*see* figure 26). Once the depth has been reached, angle the fingers slightly medially and you should feel the psoas. Direct the subject into hip flexion and you will feel the muscle shortening to confirm your location. If this is too uncomfortable, release the pressure slightly. Following this, maintain your lock and instruct the subject to straighten the leg for STR. Good release also occurs from instructing the subject into a posterior pelvic tilt. You are only really affecting the surface of this deep muscle but by locking the fascia you are incurring a release in the muscle as a whole.

Keep the subject in the same position to work the iliacus. Slowly glide over the anterior superior iliac spine and move over the concavity of the ilium. Lock and instruct your subject to straighten his leg.

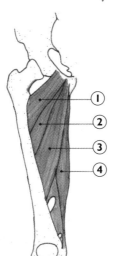

1. Pectineus
2. Adductor brevis
3. Adductor longus
4. Adductor magnus

Figure 27: Adductors.

Hip Adduction

Major Muscles: Adductor longus, adductor magnus (oblique fibres), adductor brevis, gracilis and pectineus.

All the adductors are important in preventing overbalancing laterally by keeping the thigh pulled inward during the support phase of walking and running. Tears in the adductor group are frequently termed as 'groin strain' and commonly occur when the adductors are weak in relation to the quadriceps. Sports involved with sprinting or sudden changes of direction are predisposed to this type of injury. Over-use resulting in hypertonicity such as horse riding or football can also induce problems here. Injury often presents at the muscle origin or at the musculotendinous junction. Maintenance massage is a key to gaining and maintaining flexibility and strength in the area. The adductor magnus is the largest and most posterior of the adductors. Its origin is close to the hamstrings and the muscle does assist in hip extension. Often when athletes perceive niggling 'hamstring pain' this muscle is the cause. Depending on the position of the thigh it is also involved with medial or lateral rotation.

Hip Adductors – Treatment

This is frequently a sensitive area to treat even on flexible people. It is important to ensure relaxation and this may mean significantly shortening the muscle prior to locking in. In supine position, hold the flexed knee while the foot is resting on the table. Apply pressures with the other hand at points in the muscle and on the borders of the adductor longus and the pectineus. Passively abduct the leg or guide the subject to abduct his leg into your hand making sure that the opposing hip does not rise (*see* figure 29). For the gracilis, a straight leg stretch may be more effective as the muscle also crosses the knee (*see* figure 28).

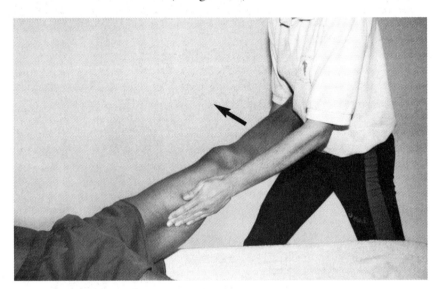

Figure 28: Pressure in the adductor longus as the therapist abducts the straight leg.

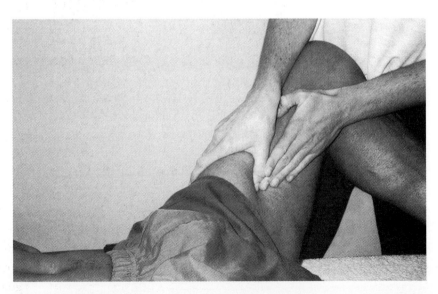

Figure 29: Pressure in the adductor longus as the subject abducts his hip.

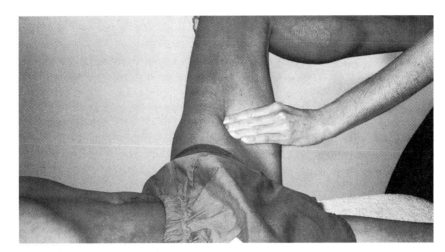

Figure 30: With the subject's foot resting on the hip of the therapist, the knee is secured for the subject to push into as pressure is applied in the adductor longus.

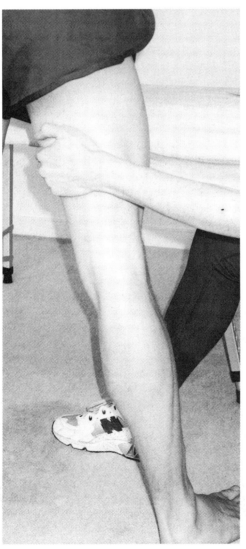

Figure 31: STR to the adductor magnus in a weight-bearing position.

To locate the adductor magnus more easily and to accommodate its role as a hip extensor, hold the flexed knee and rest the foot or lower leg on your hips for a secure hold. Apply an appropriate lock and advise the subject to abduct or flex the hip as necessary to separate adherence. The other adductors can be treated well in this position too, traversing and separating them from each other, subtly changing the movement as necessary depending on the adductor's secondary movements (*see* figure 30). Work close to the pubic bone to ensure that the origins are attended to.

Adductor magnus reacts well to weight-bearing STR, where the subject can be instructed to produce a stretch while standing (*see* figure 31).

Hip Abduction

Major Muscles: Gluteus medius, gluteus minimus, TFL, sartorius and piriformis (in the seated position).

The gluteus medius and minimus support and control the hip and pelvic tilt, through eccentric contraction, as the body weight is transferred from foot to foot during walking and running. While one foot is off the ground, contraction prevents the opposing hip from sagging. Hopping is a good exercise for the abductors.

Tensor Fasciae Latae (TFL) and Iliotibial Band (ITB)

The TFL assists in hip flexion, abduction and is a powerful medial rotator when the hip is extended. It is also a weak extensor and lateral rotator of the knee. The TFL aids stability of the hip and aids stability of the femur on the tibia in weight-bearing activities. The TFL with the gluteus maximus runs into a thick band of connective tissue known as the iliotibial band (ITB) which links the pelvis with the tibia. The ITB helps to stabilise the extended knee. If hypertonicity of the TFL develops and the ITB becomes shortened, restriction between it and the vastus lateralis can occur causing the band to rub on the lateral femoral condyle or over the greater trochanter.

When tight, this is a particularly difficult muscle and tendon to stretch free, but precise usage of STR can effectively free even severely fibrosed areas. Problems here are associated with gluteus medius hypertonicity or weakness, poor pelvic posture, tension in the vastus lateralis and weakness in the adductors.

Hip Abductors and ITB – Treatment

Side lie the subject, secure his flexed knee and abduct the hip. Apply pressure away from the iliac crest and adduct the hip. Elbows are often necessary here in cases of severe tension or fibrosity, or just a heavy leg (*see* figure 32). To avoid holding the leg, position a pillow under his knee for him to actively adduct into as the pressure is applied.

Treat the TFL side lying, as with the abductors and the superficial hip flexors. Lock in with the heel of the hand or an elbow and adduct the leg; alternatively lock and instruct the subject into a small amount of hip

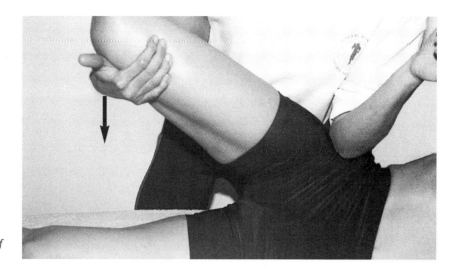

Figure 32: Use of the elbow in the gluteus medius while the subject adducts into the hand of the therapist.

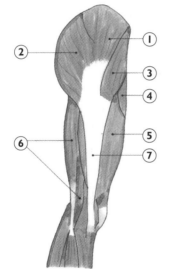

1. Gluteus medius
2. Gluteus maximus
3. Tensor fasciae latae
4. Rectus femoris
5. Vastus lateralis
6. Biceps femoris
7. Iliotibial band (ITB)

Figure 33: Lateral thigh.

extension. This area can be very sensitive and uncomfortable or even ticklish so work precisely and efficiently. The fascia can be softened by applying a CTM lock across the ITB, whilst the subject flexes or extends his hip away from the angle of pressure, still from a side lying position (*see* figure 34). Specific locks between it and the vastus lateralis anterior and posterior are essential. In this instance, the subject can flex the knee.

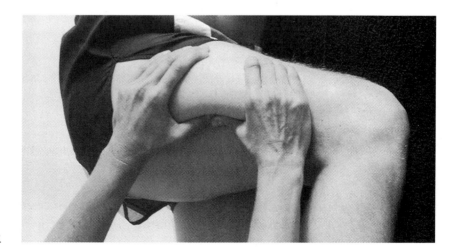

Figure 34: Pressure is attained posterior to the ITB while the subject extends the hip to stretch the fascia over the band.

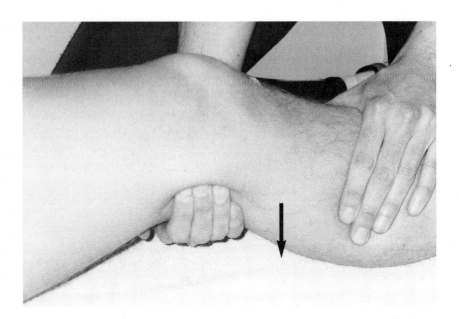

Figure 35: Locking into the tendons behind the knee as the subject extends the knee.

THE KNEE

The knee has a good range of movement. It is made stable by strong ligaments and certain musculotendinous structures, in particular: the iliotibial band, sartorius, gracilis, semimembranosus, semitendinosus, popliteus and the quadriceps. The knee is constantly under stress as weight is transferred from the body to the ground in running and walking. Over-use can develop and the knee is vulnerable to traumatic injury from twisting and turning.

The quadriceps insert into the base of the patella and the ligamentum patella then joins the patella to the tibial tuberosity. Functionally the ligamentum patella behaves as a tendon, transmitting the force of the quadriceps to the tibia, so is often referred to as the 'patella tendon'. There is a band of retaining connective tissue across the knee that is known as the patellar retinaculum.

Knee Flexion

Major Muscles: Hamstrings, gastrocnemius, gracilis, sartorius, popliteus and plantaris.

All of these muscles cross over two joints except for the popliteus. The knee flexors control extension to prevent hyperextension of the knee

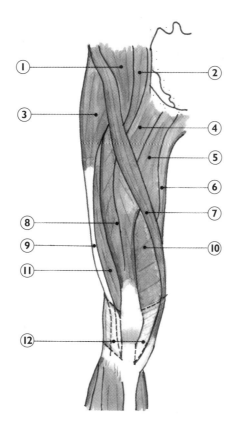

1. Iliacus
2. Psoas
3. Tensor fasciae latae
4. Pectineus
5. Adductor longus
6. Gracilis
7. Sartorius
8. Rectus femoris
9. Iliotibial band (ITB)
10. Vastus medialis
11. Vastus lateralis
12. Patellar retinaculum

Figure 36: Anterior thigh – quadriceps, adductors and hip flexors.

during walking and standing. Pain behind the knee can be due to any of these muscles being tight, often the hamstrings. Commonly they can be strained through running, kicking or dancing. Congestion in the sartorius and gracilis can cause medial knee pain, but it is important that all of the tendons around the knee are treated as well as the entire muscle. STR to the popliteus, the tendons of insertion to the hamstrings, gracilis and sartorius, and the tendons of origin for the gastrocnemius.

Knee Flexors – Treatment

With the subject in prone position and the knee flexed, apply the lock and straighten the knee; apply STR to the three hamstring muscles separating and releasing any adherence (*see* page 37). Progress to the tendons of

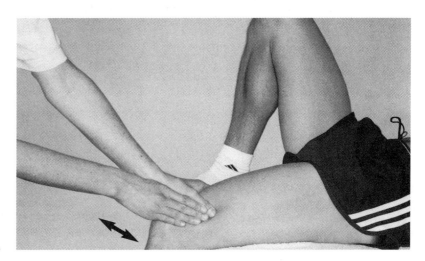

Figure 37: STR to the quadriceps.

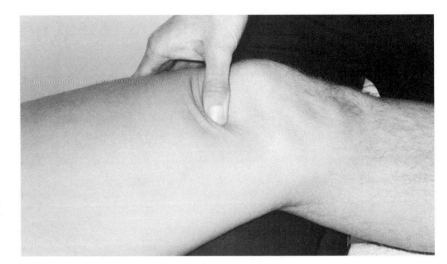

Figure 38: The knee is extended to shorten the muscle and pressure is applied in the vastus medialis away from the knee as the therapist flexes it.

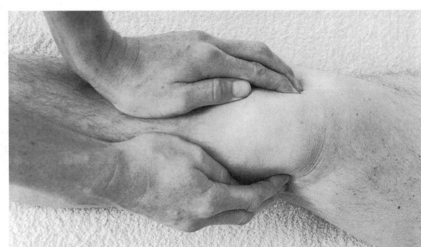

Figure 39: Pressure away from the patella to stretch the retinaculum as the subject flexes the knee.

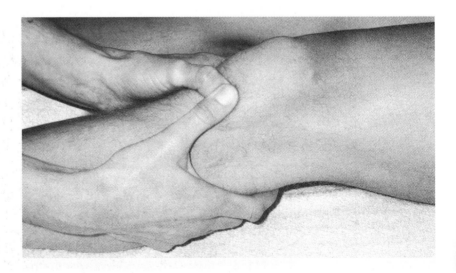

Figure 40: Pressure across the patellar tendon as the subject flexes the knee.

insertion of the hamstrings, gastrocnemius, gracilis and sartorius. Alternatively, with the subject in supine position and the knee slightly flexed, lock into the tendons with the fingers and maintain each pressure while the subject extends or flattens his knee into the lock provided (*see* figure 35). The gastrocnemius is primarily released with the other plantar flexors, the gracilis with the adductors and the sartorius as a whole with the hip flexors.

Knee Extension

Major Muscles: Quadriceps group: rectus femoris, vastus lateralis, vastus medialis (including oblique) and vastus intermedius.

The rectus femoris works strongly as a knee extensor when the hip is extended and is ineffective when the hip is flexed. The vastus medialis is strong in the final stages of knee extension. The TFL is also a very weak knee extensor.

The quadriceps is a powerful muscle group, and is exercised significantly in walking, running and jumping. The rectus femoris goes over two joints (it is also involved with hip flexion) so is more susceptible to strain. Separating and localised stretching will help to rebalance the four muscles and ensure that full function and strength are maintained minimising the possibility of impairment or breakdown to the quadriceps but also preventing over-use injuries to the knee. There is a danger in working too early on the quadriceps after a direct trauma in that the formation of myositis ossificans is a possibility.

Knee Extensors – Treatment

With the subject supine, support his knee in a semi-flexed position. Extend the knee, apply a lock and flex the knee (*see* figure 38). For a more effective stretch, the subject lies on his back with the leg to be worked on over the end of the table and the other leg flexed at the hip to protect the back (*see* figure 37). Apply pressures towards the origins and slightly transversely to the fibres to separate the vastus lateralis from adherence to the ITB, and the vastus medialis from the sartorius and the adductors. The stretch in these instances is best achieved with the subject actively flexing the knee. Side lying is a good way to work on the rectus femoris by taking the hip into extension (*see* figure 25) and the position is also good for achieving separation of the vastus lateralis from the ITB with active knee flexion.

Knee Problems

There are particular knee injuries that benefit from STR work. Patella tracking problems can be helped by ensuring all of the quadriceps are separate. By relieving adhesion and tension in the lateral thigh and ITB, treatment may facilitate efficient strength gains in the vastus medialis. This will enable re-balance to occur. In the case of a synovial plica, in conjunction with traditional friction techniques, STR of both medial and lateral retinaculum around the knee will break fibrous tissue and stretch and nourish the surrounding connective tissue. Specific STR to the medial ligament complex, in the event of injury, is beneficial. General work to the quadriceps will relieve stress placed on the knee in tendonitis problems. Specific minimal STR on the patellar tendon itself will divide adhesive tissue there. In Osgood-Schlatter's syndrome, treatment of the insertion point should be avoided, but the quadriceps need to be released from their hypertonicity and STR will provide valuable relief. ITB syndrome can be treated where the band itself is tight and the commonly associated adherence between it and the vastus lateralis (*see* page 44). With this condition, congestion in the lateral retinaculum must also be considered. Post surgery conditions quickly benefit from active STR, where muscles are atrophied and range of movement has been reduced. It is useful in that the subject can control his range of stretch and the muscles and fascia may be released of fibrous tissue so that efficient strength gains can be attained.

Knee – Treatment

Systematically apply CTM locks at points away from the medial and lateral border of the patella as the subject flexes his knee (*see* figure 39). Attention is necessary at fibrous areas but it is important to glide into the lock slowly and precisely as this may be particularly sensitive. Treatment of the medial ligament is possible with the same procedure. When treating the patellar tendon, a transverse lock to stretch the tendon sheath, needs to be applied as the subject is guided into knee flexion (*see* figure 40).

It is possible to treat the knee with the subject weight-bearing. With the subject standing, lock in on either side of the patella to affect the medial and lateral retinaculum and guide him into a squat. This dynamic treatment may have quick positive results for patellar-tracking problems (*see* figure 41).

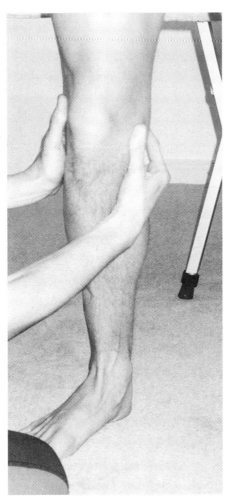

Figure 41: STR to the connective tissues away from the patella in a weight-bearing position.

Plantar Flexion

Major Muscles: **Superficial compartment**: Gastrocnemius, soleus and plantaris. **Deep compartment**: Tibialis posterior, flexor digitorum longus and flexor hallucis longus. **Lateral compartment**: Peroneus longus and peroneus brevis.

The gastrocnemius and soleus are the primary plantar flexors of the ankle. During the push off phase in vigorous walking and running the gastrocnemius is one of the most powerful muscles in the body and the tendo calcaneus (Achilles tendon) which forms the insertion point for both muscles is very thick and strong. The soleus also contracts statically to maintain stance. As well as plantar flexion, the gastrocnemius flexes the knee and because it crosses over two joints is more susceptible to strain. Many over-use problems arise in the lower leg. Imbalances can occur. For example, if the gastrocnemius is stretched well with a straight leg stretch and the soleus due to its attachment below the knee is not stretched out fully with a bent knee stretch, then adherence of these two muscles can develop. Congestion frequently manifests at the musculotendinous junction. Compartment syndromes can prevail where imbalance occurs.

Plantar Flexors – Treatment

Treat the calf generally with STR. Tension and adhesive tissue quickly become evident. With the subject supine and the leg straight, lock in between the bellies of the gastrocnemius and instruct him to dorsiflex the foot (*see* figure 42).

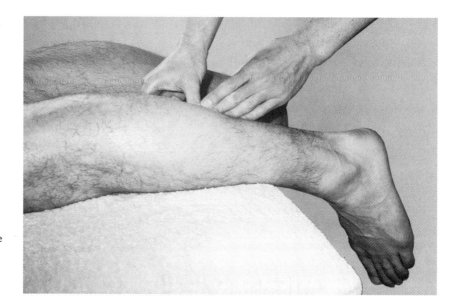

Figure 42: Pressure between the bellies of the gastrocnemius as the subject dorsiflexes the foot.

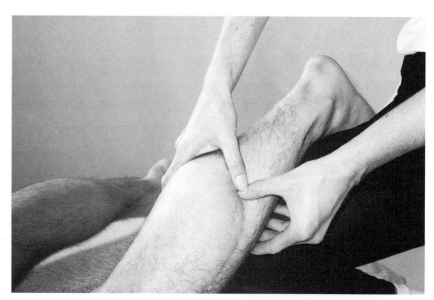

Figure 43: Pressure between the gastrocnemius and the soleus as the subject dorsiflexes the foot.

Systematically work the lateral and medial aspects of the muscle. With the knee flexed and the lower leg resting on your thigh, deeper and more specific work can be administered (*see* figure 43). The lock can be angled to separate the soleus and gastrocnemius adherence from the lateral or the medial border. This can be conducted by working up from the musculotendinous junction. Application of a deeper pressure, once the gastrocnemius and soleus have been treated, will release the deep posterior compartment. Locking can also be conducted by hooking away from the tibia in this same flexed knee position to release congestion by the bone.

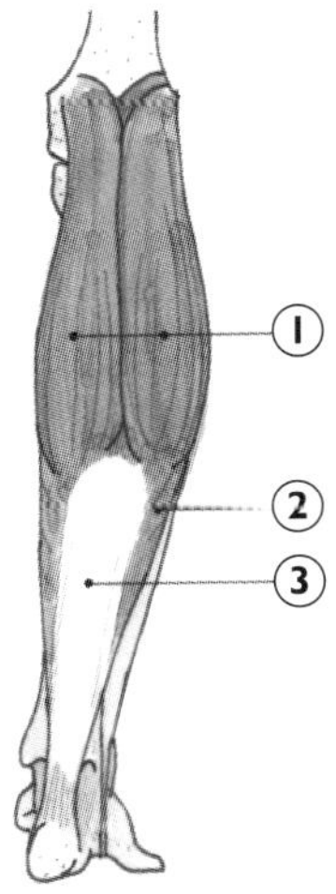

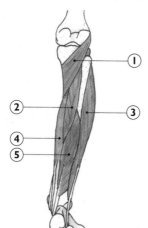

1. Gastrocnemius
2. Soleus
3. Tendo calcaneus
   (Achilles tendon)

Figure 44:
Superficial calf muscles.

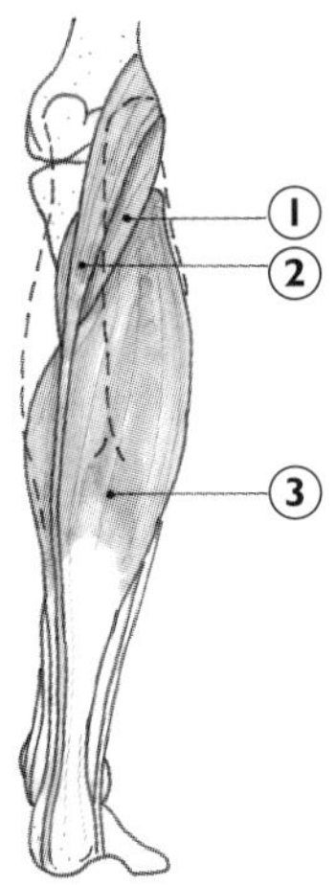

1. Popliteus
2. Plantaris
3. Soleus

Figure 45:
Deep calf muscles.

1. Popliteus
2. Tibialis posterior
3. Peroneus longus
4. Flexor digitorum longus
5. Flexor hallucis longus

Figure 46:
Deep calf muscles II.

Achilles Tendon

Achilles tendinitis or peritendinitis can become chronic as a result of over-use. The causative activity needs to be moderated, or stopped, as the condition can become easily aggravated. A general calf treatment is important as congestion in the gastrocnemius and soleus can often be the reason for problems in the Achilles.

Following this, gently pinch the tendon. Lift the paratenon from the tendon and ask the client to dorsiflex the foot (*see* figure 48). Treat like this working from the calcaneus to the musculotendinous junction in the calf.

STR following surgery from Achilles partial or complete rupture works well as part of rehabilitation. Apply STR to the lower leg as a whole, including the foot, and treat the Achilles as just mentioned.

Dorsiflexion

Major Muscles: Tibialis anterior, extensor digitorum longus, extensor hallucis longus and peroneus tertius (not always present).

The tibialis anterior is the main dorsi flexor. Posturally, it is important to maintain balance as the distribution of weight changes. It also controls foot plant. The extensor digitorum longus plays a role in maintaining balance between plantar and dorsiflexion. The fascia is thick in the anterior lower leg so there is a higher risk of sustaining compartment syndrome type injuries due to over training. This could be a sudden increase in exercise particularly on hard surfaces such as exercise classes, a build up of running mileage or walking too far in unaccustomed heavy shoes. The anterior compartment becomes tight and the fascial covering tense, causing a pressure between it and the muscle. Ultimately, the pressure can cause restricted blood supply, pain and loss of function. Rest is essential in the acute stages.

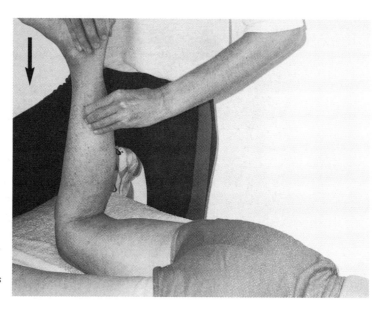

Figure 47: Pressure in the calves as the therapist dorsiflexes the foot.

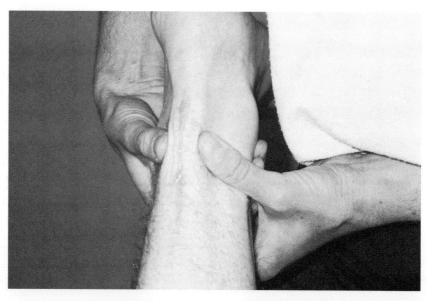

Figure 48: Locking on either side of the Achilles tendon to stretch the fascia as the subject dorsiflexes the foot.

Dorsi Flexors – Treatment

STR using a CTM lock is effective at reducing this pressure build-up. Lock in to forcefully stretch the fascia towards the points of origin and maintain the hold while the underlying muscles are momentarily elongated with active plantar flexion (*see* figure 49). Work from the ankle up the shin, then return and separate the tendons under the retinaculum. STR will cause minimal aggravation and will manage the problem. Even in severe cases it could prevent the need for a fasciotomy.

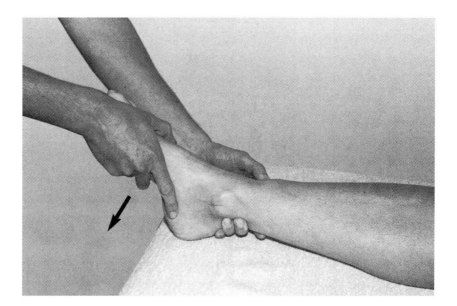

Figure 49: Pressure in the tibialis anterior as the foot is plantar flexed.

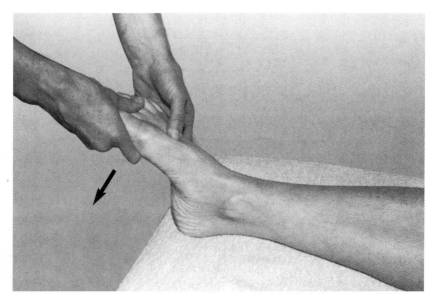

Figure 50: Pressure between the extensor tendons over the foot as the toes are flexed.

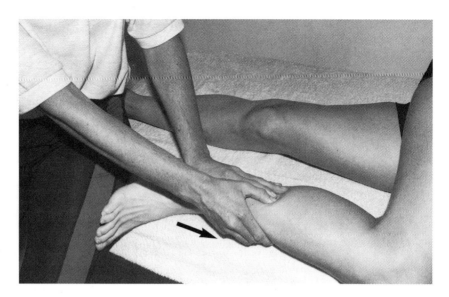

Figure 51: Pressure in the peroneus longus as the foot is dorsiflexed.

Inversion of Foot

Major Muscles: Tibialis posterior, tibialis anterior, flexor digitorum longus, flexor hallucis longus and extensor hallucis longus.

The tibialis posterior helps maintain and control forefoot positioning, by preventing the medial arch from flattening. Its tendon attachments are palpable at the medial malleolus and the navicular. Tenosynovitis can occur with over-use.

Eversion of Foot

Major Muscles: Peroneus longus, peroneus brevis and peroneus tertius (not always present).

Peroneus longus contributes to posture by helping to maintain the medial arch. The brevis aids the maintenance of the longitudinal arch. The peroneal muscles have a major function in controlling ankle stability on rough terrain.

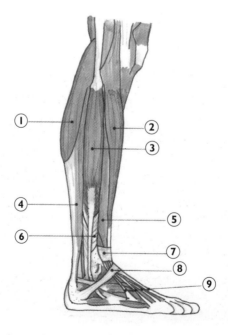

1. Gastrocnemius
2. Tibialis anterior
3. Peroneus longus
4. Tendo calcaneus
   (Achilles tendon)
5. Extensor digitorum longus
6. Peroneus brevis
7. Superior extensor
   retinaculum
8. Inferior extensor retinaculum
9. Extensor digitorum longus

Figure 52: Lateral lower leg.

Invertors and Evertors – Treatment

With the subject supine, hook under the peroneus longus at the lateral malleolus and maintain the lock until the client has inverted and/or dorsiflexed his foot. Follow the muscle up the side of the leg. Treatment can also take place effectively in side lying position (*see* figure 51). The brevis can be located around the lateral ankle and is a prime muscle to consider in ankle inversion sprains.

THE ANKLE

General work to the lower leg and foot needs to be undertaken with the presentation of any ankle problem. STR in these muscles is highly beneficial following ankle sprains. It can be used directly following RICE during the general rehabilitative measures, to ensure strength gains. It is also useful in the instance of a poorly healed ankle presenting with weakness and instability due to fibrous tissue and imbalance, even many years after the initial injury. Inversion sprains are the most common ankle sprains, affecting the anterior and posterior talofibular ligament and the calcanofibular ligament and/or the peronei. Following the sprain, adherence commonly occurs within the extensor tendon sheaths, the extensor retinaculum and ligaments, hence leaving a residual egg-shaped swelling. In this instance STR on the ligament is useful together with work

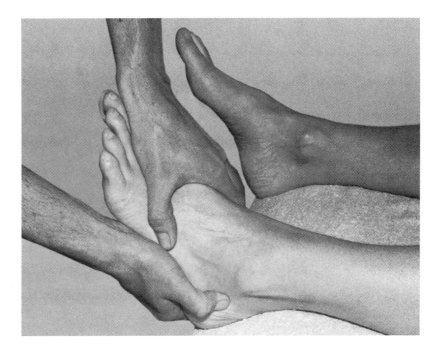

Figure 53: A CTM lock is attained away from the lateral malleolus as the subject dorsiflexes the foot.

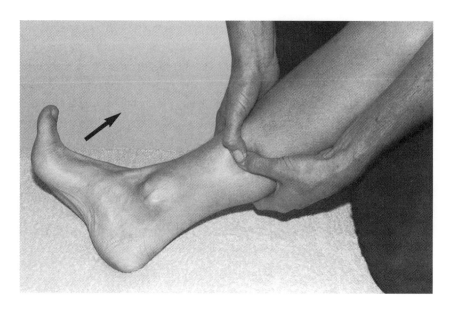

Figure 54: Pressure away from the medial border of the tibia as the foot is dorsiflexed.

on all the everting and dorsiflexing muscles. Balance still needs to be restored wherever the primary damage is, so locking on to ligamentous tissue as well as on and between the tendons, and instructing an appropriate stretch is effective in restoring freedom of movement. Combination movements of flexion, extension, eversion and inversion work well in separating the tendons from each other and from the retinaculum, as they take in all the primary and secondary movements of the muscles.

Once the ankle is moving well, strength training and proprioceptive re-education exercises become more effective and permanent. In the case of major injury such as ligamentous rupture or bone breakage, healing will always be slow. Swelling, scar tissue, pain and reduced movement can become permanent due to the damage and forced immobilisation; STR, as outlined above, will prove invaluable in regaining ankle mobility and in reducing swelling.

Shin Splints

This is a general term for chronic pain in the lower leg. It can arise from the anterior, posterior and sometimes the lateral compartment, although more commonly it refers to pain occurring on the medial tibial border. This is known as 'medial tibial stress syndrome'.

Specific to pain on the medial tibial border, the plantar flexors require particular attention. Chronic problems are usually caused by the soleus, flexor digitorum longus and tibialis posterior, and frequently present in the lower third of the tibia. The injury can be due to hypertonicity or compartment syndrome of the muscle, adhesion between the tendon and the bone, inflammation of the periosteum or an actual stress fracture of the bone. Many distance runners who suffer with this condition successfully resort to prescribed orthotics. The repetitive nature of the sport can make a minor biomechanical deficiency apparent. Whether orthotics are necessary or not, soft tissue release is an indispensable form of treatment for shin splints. STR will decrease tissue adherence and tension with minimal aggravation to the inflammation.

Shin Splints – Treatment

Wherever the pain presents, it is imperative to treat the whole lower leg and foot. Progress to the deeper flexor muscles, once the gastrocnemius and soleus have been softened. Glide a thumb or fingers medially off of the tibia, lock still and dorsiflex the foot (*see* figure 54). If there is major discomfort or concern of a stress fracture, remember to conduct the seven second test (*see* page 19) to ensure that treatment is only administered around and not on an inflamed area. It is necessary to treat the foot thoroughly to relieve congestion within the insertion tendons and plantar fascia.

THE FOOT

The foot is a vital area to maintain. Strong, flexible musculature will enhance its shock absorbency minimising the risk of injury. Control and good movement of the joints in the foot are possible where the soft tissues

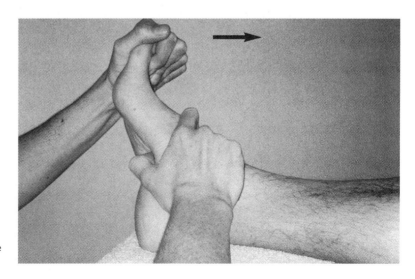

Figure 55: Pressure with the thumb in the plantar fascia while the therapist extends the toes.

are strong and supple. All this encourages efficient and correct foot plant and reduces the possibility of repercussions elsewhere. Whilst standing still, the arches of the foot are maintained primarily by strong ligaments in the sole. There are four layers of intrinsic muscles on the plantar surface that help support the arches of the foot as well as to move the toes. These muscles, together with the long tendons that cross the ankle, maintain the arches during movement. Thick layers of connective tissue envelop the muscles and fatty tissue to provide protection for the foot.

There are many injuries which can occur in the toes such as: turf toe, which is a sprain to the first metatarso-phalangeal joint (MPJ), metatarsalgia which refers to general pain in the forefoot, hallux valgus and hallux rigidus which result from excess or lack of mobility in the MPJ. Once diagnosed, STR can be of huge benefit in relieving discomfort and can contribute to the development of good foot mechanics by restoring muscle balance.

Toe Flexion

Major Muscles: Flexor digitorum longus, flexor digitorum brevis, flexor hallucis longus, flexor hallucis brevis, flexor digiti minimi brevis, interossei, quadratus plantae and lumbricals.

Toe Flexors – Treatment

Treat the deep posterior compartment (*see* page 52) then treat the foot as with the plantar fascia (*see* figures 55 and 56).

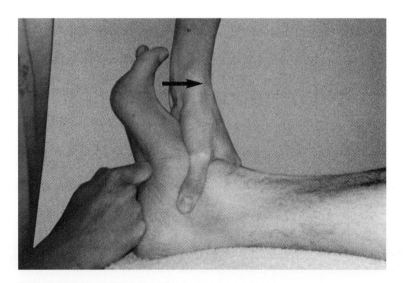

Figure 56: A deeper pressure can be attained using the knuckle as the subject extends the toes.

Toe Extension

Major Muscles: Extensor hallucis longus, extensor digitorum longus and extensor digitorum brevis, lumbricals and the interossei.

Toe Extensors – Treatment

Treat the dorsi flexors, then apply pressures over the top of the foot. Glide over and divide the extensor tendons, hold the position and flex the toes (curl them under, *see* figure 50).

Abduction

Major Muscles: Abductor hallucis, abductor digiti minimi, dorsal interossei.

Adduction

Major Muscles: Adductor hallucis, plantar interossei.

Plantar Fasciitis

The plantar aponeurosis (plantar fascia) is a very thick fibrous band of tissue in the base of the foot which covers the plantar muscles and is vital in maintaining the longitudinal arches of the foot. Over pronation of weak lateral leg muscles can predispose the plantar fascia to injury. The fascia becomes thickened and inflamed. Medial pain at its calcaneal attachment is usual in this condition as well as general tension in the base of the foot.

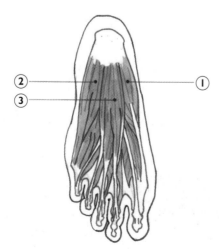

1. Abductor hallucis
2. Abductor digiti minimi
3. Flexor digitorum brevis

Figure 57: Plantar view of foot superficial muscles.

Plantar Fasciitis – Treatment

It is important to work the calf, Achilles tendon and plantar muscles. These are usually hypertonic or fibrosed if the plantar fascia is shortened. A CTM lock is needed whilst the toes are extended. Active work is essential so a strong lock can be maintained. A strong knuckle will prove a useful tool in this treatment (*see* figures 55 and 56).

Part 4
Trunk and Neck

THE SPINE

The spine consists of thirty-three individual vertebrae: seven cervical, twelve thoracic, five lumbar and the sacrum (five fused) and coccyx (four fused). Although only small movements occur between each vertebra, the combined action of all of them facilitates good overall spinal mobility. Between each vertebra is a cartilaginous disc; the discs make up approximately one third of the total height of the spine. The vertebral column is maintained in its upright posture by strong ligaments and muscles; it has three natural curves (four including the sacral curve) which together with the intervertebral discs are responsible for absorbing shock. Flexible, strong muscles will enhance the fluid content of the discs and allow for efficient maintenance of the spinal curvature.

Most people will suffer with backache at some point in their lives, although maintenance of correct posture would reduce the likelihood of injury problems. Good spinal posture places minimal strain on the muscles that maintain the body's stance. If the body sways from its neutral position, it is counteracted by muscles which contract eccentrically. If an inefficient posture is continued, then adaptive responses lead to hypertonicity in the muscles, loss of spinal mobility and dysfunction. Postural adaptation often develops over many years and people are not aware of a problem until the tension and imbalance give rise to a traumatic injury, such as a prolapsed disc.

The position of the pelvis is affected by the abdominal muscles and spinal extensors as well as the hip flexors and extensors. An increase in the lumbar

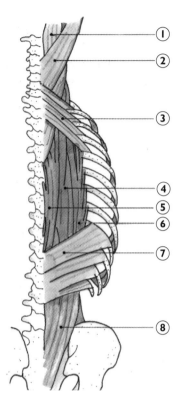

1. Semispinalis capitis
2. Splenius capitis
3. Serratus posterior superior
4. Longissimus dorsi
5. Spinalis
6. Iliocostalis
7. Serratus posterior inferior
8. Thoracolumbar fascia

Figure 58: Deep back muscles.

lordotic curve will result in tight hip flexors and back extensors, weak abdominal muscles and a tendency for compensatory thoracic kyphosis. The side flexors need to be evaluated with regard to lateral imbalance. Massage therapists need to be systematic in treating the hips and antagonists with any presentation of back pain. There are many different types of stresses placed on posture and the therapist needs to be aware if the subject suffers from any of these. There may be a structural problem, such as a leg length discrepancy. Occupational factors such as driving for long hours or sitting behind a keyboard may be involved. If sports are the cause it could be repetitiveness, as for example in long-distance cycling, or it could be the overload on one side, such as in golf or tennis. The root of the problem needs to be addressed and altered if possible. Maintenance massage of the back area is invaluable. Correct posture is still not well understood by the general public so, following treatment, postural awareness should be discussed along with stretching exercises.

Traumatic injuries sustained from heavy lifting or falling, sciatic, disc and degenerative conditions will benefit from having the soft tissues strong, supple and in balance.

Spine Extension

Major Muscles: Erector spinae: Iliocostalis, longissimus, spinalis. Quadratus lumborum, interspinales, multifidis, semispinalis and gluteus maximus from a flexed position.

When all three muscles on both sides of the erector spinae contract, it is the main extensor of the back. The iliocostalis (lateral layer) has attachments that run the length of the spine. The longissimus (middle layer) and the spinalis (medial layer) attach to the skull and to the cervical and thoracic vertebrae. There are many complex muscle contractions always occurring as the erector spinae also controls flexion of the spine and stabilises the non weight-bearing side, to prevent the pelvis from dropping during side flexion. The erector spinae is also critical in maintaining the secondary curve.

The transversospinalis muscles are found deep to the erector spinae and in order of superficial to deep are: semispinalis, multifidis, rotatores and interspinales. The deepest muscles cross only one or two vertebrae.

Spine Side Flexion

Major Muscles: Quadratus lumborum, erector spinae, intertransversarii, external oblique, internal oblique, rectus abdominis and multifidis.

Side flexion is produced by muscles on that side. When standing on one leg, the quadratus lumborum acts strongly on the non weight-bearing side to stop the pelvis from dropping. It also stabilises the twelfth rib during forced expiration by fixing the origin of the diaphragm. When both contract, they are responsible for lumbar spine extension and stability.

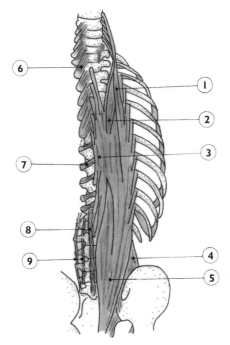

1. Iliocostalis
2. Longissimus dorsi
3. Spinalis
4. Quadratus lumborum
5. Thoracolumbar fascia
6. Multifidis
7. Rotatores
8. Interspinales
9. Intertransversarii

Figure 59: Deep back muscles II.

Spine Rotation

Major Muscles: External oblique, internal oblique, multifidis, rotatores, semispinalis.

During rotation to one side, contraction of the external oblique on the opposing side and contraction of the internal oblique on the same side occurs. The external oblique is the most superficial side muscle and its origins interrelate with the serratus anterior. The internal obliques run diagonally in the opposite direction.

Fascia of the Trunk

The trunk, like the rest of the body, is covered with superficial and deep fascia. The deep fascia of the neck area is thick and strong, enveloping the muscles, supporting and connecting the trunk to the muscles of the shoulder girdle and upper limb. There is a specialised deep layer of fascia in the lower back known as the thoracolumbar fascia. It consists of three layers located in the lower thoracic, lumbar and sacral, regions. The posterior layer is superficial to the erector spinae and the latissimus dorsi partially arises from it. The middle layer is between the erector spinae and the quadratus lumborum and the anterior and thinnest of the layers is located in front of the quadratus lumborum. All three converge together at the lateral border of the erector spinae. This then extends to form an origin for the transversus abdominis and internal oblique.

CTM locks are very beneficial in ensuring that the muscle can regain full separation. As many of the lower back muscles in particular are so strong, the quality of the lock is crucial for any release to occur.

The deep fascia of the abdomen is thin and elastic to allow for chest and abdomen expansion. The lower abdomen consists of aponeurosis (external oblique) and membrane.

Extensors and Side Flexors – Treatment

With the subject in a side lying position, make a secure reinforced lock just above the sacroiliac joint close to the spine and instruct him into a

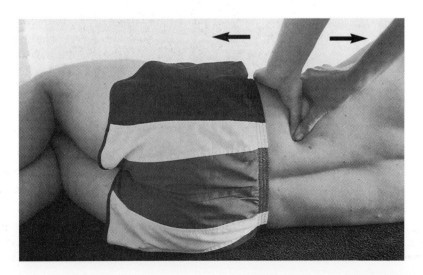

Figure 60: Pressure in the quadratus lumborum as the subject extends the hip and abducts the shoulder.

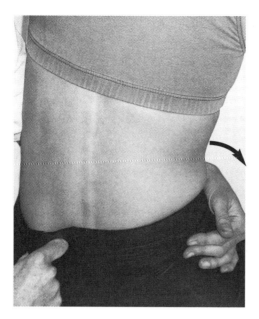

Figure 61: A CTM lock away from the vertebrae as the subject side flexes, to affect a 'release' in the thoracolumbar fascia.

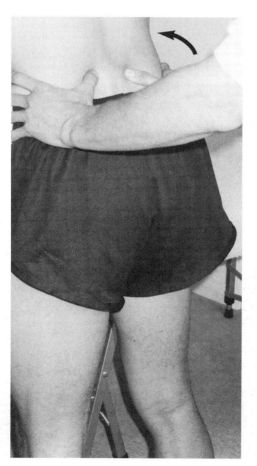

Figure 62: STR to the lower back in a weight-bearing position.

posterior tilt of the pelvis. The pressure should be directed slightly towards the head. The pelvic tilt provides a small stretch but the movement is controlled and precise. Trunk flexion can be used but the movement may prove too severe for a lock to be maintained. Apply pressure and move up the whole of the lumbar area then return and treat more laterally to the initial locks. Treat around the sacroiliac joint with two or three CTM locks and either a pelvic tilt, or flexion of the spine or hip (*see* figure 15). For the quadratus lumborum, take the depth of the erector spinae muscle and drop in on the lateral border of the muscle. Maintain this pressure while the subject extends the hip and abducts the arm (*see* figure 60).

Treatment of the erector spinae can continue until it reaches an area not affected by the stretch from the pelvic movement. This procedure is usually only beneficial around the lumbar area. For 'release' in the erector spinae muscles further up the back it will be necessary to lock as the subject flexes the trunk. The direction of pressure in this case should be towards the base of the trunk.

Weight-bearing STR on occasion may prove to be a useful technique. With the subject standing and supporting himself on the treatment table or wall, apply a CTM lock and instruct him into flexion or side flexion of the spine (*see* figure 62).

Seated STR works well even on the larger individual. As the muscles are under tension it is advised to treat the top layer of the thoracolumbar fascia rather than trying to delve into the strength of the extensors. By applying a CTM lock, whilst securing the subject across the front of the hips, and instructing him to side flex or rotate, severe muscle shortening can be relieved because of the fascial release (*see* figure 61). By having the arm raised on the side being treated, the stretch on the latissimus dorsi may enhance the STR effect. Also, with the subject seated, the quadratus lumborum can be targeted and the subject can side flex (*see* figure 63).

Spine Flexion

Major Muscles: Rectus abdominis, external oblique, internal oblique, psoas major and minor (when the insertions are fixed).

Flexion occurs during concentric contraction of the muscles on both sides. The flexors also affect the position of the pelvis by affecting its tilt and subsequently the curvature of the lumbar spine. Attachments of the abdominal muscles on the pelvis, at the pubis symphysis and muscles within the abdominal wall are all occasionally torn, and fascial adherence

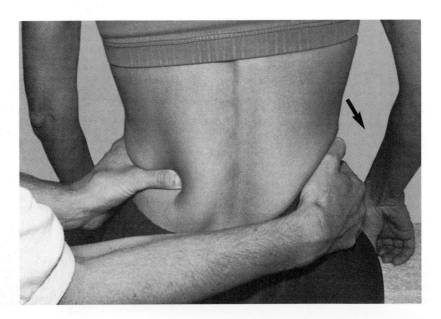

Figure 63: Pressure in the quadratus lumborum as the subject side flexes.

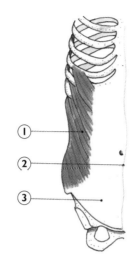

1. External oblique
2. Linea alba
3. Fascia

Figure 64: Anterior abdomen – superficial muscles.

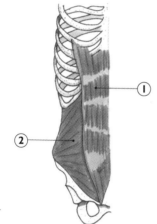

1. Rectus abdominis
2. Internal oblique

Figure 65: Anterior abdomen – deep muscles.

can develop. Thickening of the fascia can occur with poor posture leading to further postural imbalance and weakness. If the muscles are weak, the pelvis is dropped, the hip flexors and spine extensors in relation become hypertonic, and the lumbar curve tends towards lordosis. Correct, isolated strengthening of the abdominal muscles is necessary to regain lost strength.

Spine Flexors and Rotators – Treatment

Position the subject supine. When treating the rectus abdominis, start from the origin on the pubis with a CTM lock and advise the subject into a very minimal side flexion. Progress to the outer borders of the muscle, on one side, hooking under it while he side flexes (*see* figure 66). Angle the lock carefully near to the insertions to avoid bruising from the bone. Check the section on hip flexors for treatment of the psoas (*see* page 39). The external and internal obliques may be treated in a similar fashion, by applying pressure as the subject side flexes. It is also possible to treat the oblique muscles in a side lying position where a small rotational movement may provide adequate stretch for a release. Locks must be applied away from the movement and pressure should be angled to produce a shallow CTM lock.

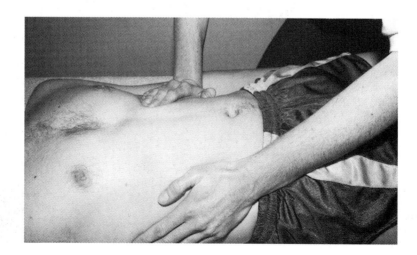

Figure 66: Pressure in the lateral border of the rectus abdominis as the subject side flexes.

Compression of Abdomen

Major Muscles: Transversus abdominis, external oblique, internal oblique and rectus abdominis.

These muscles increase abdominal pressure and provide a muscular support for the pelvis, abdomen and viscera.

RESPIRATION

Inspiration

Major Muscles: Diaphragm, external intercostals, levatores costarum, serratus posterior and superior, pectoralis minor, sternocleidomastoid.

Expiration

Major Muscles: Transversus abdominis, subcostales, transversus thoracis, internal intercostals, external oblique, internal oblique, latissimus dorsi and quadratus lumborum (fixes ribs).

The diaphragm is a large sheet of muscle that separates the thoracic and abdominal cavities. As it contracts it is drawn downwards and the subsequent change in pressure causes air at atmospheric pressure to enter the lungs. When it relaxes, it returns to its initial position and air is expelled from the lungs. During forced expiration, i.e. during moderate or heavy exercise, the expiratory muscles become involved to drive air out more quickly. Through their contraction, there is an increase in abdominal

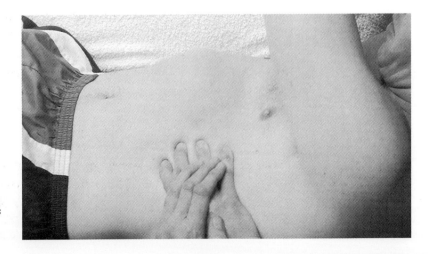

Figure 67: Pressure between the ribs in the intercostal muscles as the subject breathes in deeply and exhales.

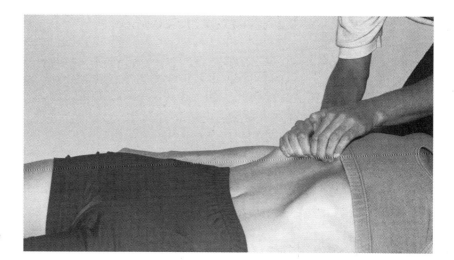

Figure 68: Pressure towards the diaphragm with the fingers.

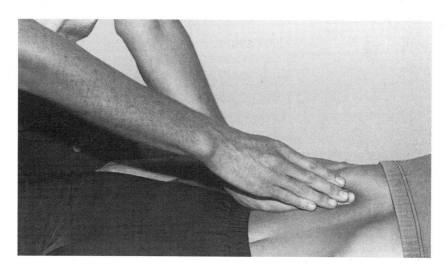

Figure 69: Pressure under the lower ribs towards the diaphragm with the thumb and fingers as the subject breathes in slowly and deeply and exhales.

pressure that pushes the diaphragm up quicker to expel air faster. The transversus abdominis (the deepest of the abdominal muscles) is the most powerful expiratory muscle. The internal and external intercostal muscles crisscross the ribs and are responsible for drawing the ribs together (for expiration) and apart (for inspiration) respectively.

Respiratory Muscles – Treatment

Treatment of the respiratory muscles is beneficial for anyone who suffers with breathing difficulties. STR will have a positive effect on asthma sufferers. Athletes will find it can improve their breathing technique as their chest adopts a new lightness and freedom.

Ensure that the subject is in a comfortable supine position with his knees and hips bent. Gently guide a thumb behind and in front of the lower ribs towards the anterior attachments of the diaphragm whilst the subject is slowly inhaling. Hold the position and allow him to finish inhaling. Still maintaining the pressure, instruct him to exhale gently. Release the pressure (*see* figures 68 and 69). For the intercostals, side lying position is a good way of exposing the ribs. Lock in between the ribs, hold the pressure and instruct the subject to breathe in and to breathe out (*see* figure 67). The external intercostals are the most superficial and, therefore, affected more directly from this technique.

THE NECK

Neck flexors are generally weaker than the extensors that have to hold the heavy head in an upright position, against gravity. The extensors are constantly under tension, contracting statically and eccentrically to maintain posture. Postural deficiencies can occur especially with repetitive activities or positions such as sitting, writing for long periods, painting a ceiling, or sporting pursuits such as cycling. The soft tissues can become micro torn and tense and, as the activity persists, holding patterns and imbalances prevail. An increase in the cervical curve, forcing the head forwards, is a common result. Problems manifest as movement restrictions, muscle, joint and nerve pain, headaches, vertigo and tinnitus. Impingement of vertebral arteries and nerves can occur which are not necessarily muscular in source and medical advice needs to be sought if presenting with referred pain or dizziness. As well as their specific movements, many of the small neck muscles are involved with maintaining balance and stability of the head on the neck; these you cannot palpate, so they will not be discussed. The platysma is the most superficial anterior muscle and is a thin flat muscle that adheres to the skin.

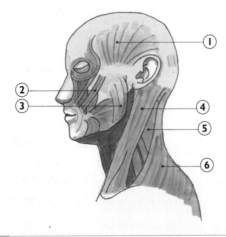

1. Temporalis
2. Zygomaticus major
3. Masseter
4. Sternocleidomastoid
5. Splenius capitis
6. Trapezius

Figure 70: Neck.

General work of all the neck muscles, systematically working the agonists and antagonists will ensure good recovery of chronic neck tension and side-effects such as headaches. It will also facilitate a return to good posture and enhanced functioning capacity.

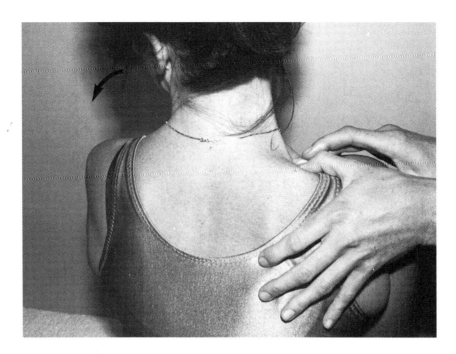

Figure 71: Treatment of the upper fibres of the trapezius with pressure as the neck is flexed or side flexed.

Due to its extreme mobility, the neck is also vulnerable to traumatic injury, one example being whiplash. Following such injury, there will be ligamentous damage and the neck muscles will present with extreme tension. This is due to fierce reflex muscle contractions that protect the head against rapid movement. Providing that medical screening is satisfactory, STR is an indispensable therapy. Degenerative conditions in the neck also benefit from soft tissue work as strong supple muscle will relieve pressure from the vertebrae and discs.

Neck Flexion

Major Muscles: The sternocleidomastoid (SCM), scalenus anterior and longus colli flex the neck. The longus capitis and SCM flex the neck and head. The rectus capitis anterior flexes the head on the neck and stabilises the atlanto-occipital joint.

Neck Side Flexion

Major Muscles: The scalenus anterior, scalenus medius and scalenus posterior, splenius cervicis, levator scapulae and SCM side flex the neck. The SCM, splenius capitis, trapezius and erector spinae side flex the head and neck. The rectus capitis lateralis side flexes the head on the neck.

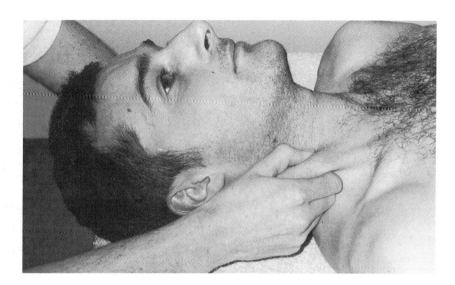

Figure 72: Pressure on either side of the SCM as the neck is side flexed or rotated.

With the sternocleidomastoid (SCM), flexion occurs when both sides contract, and side flexion to the same side or rotation to the opposite side when one side contracts. When the head and neck are fixed, the SCM can raise the clavicles and sternum therefore assisting in inspiration. The scaleni also, when contracting bilaterally, assist in neck flexion and if one side only contracts they assist in side flexion to the same side. The brachial plexus runs between the scalenus anterior and the scalenus medius.

Neck Flexors and Side Flexors – Treatment

With the subject in supine position, support the head with one hand and gently grasp the SCM with the other hand. Maintain this hold and

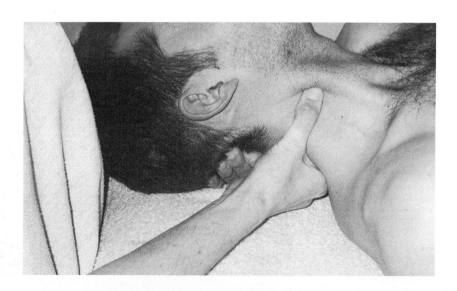

Figure 73: Pressure to the lateral side of the SCM as the neck is rotated to the same side.

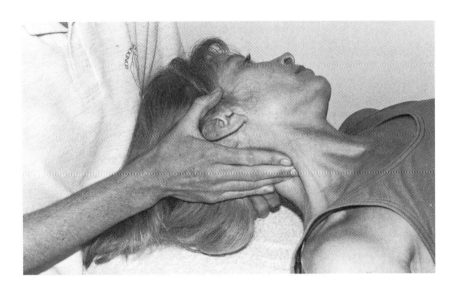

Figure 74: Pressure in the trapezius as the subject side flexes.

carefully move the neck away from this lock into side flexion to the opposite side or rotation to the same side (*see* figure 72). It is vital not to move too quickly. If the area is particularly congested, apply pressure to one side of the muscle at a time. Lock into the attachments of origin, moving to two or three new points to free the clavicular and sternal fibres (*see* figure 73). STR at the insertion points of the SCM, at the skull, is needed and a CTM lock will prove highly successful where fascial thickening is often evident; use of the knuckle away from the bone is helpful in attaining a lock but move carefully into position. The anterior scalenus can be treated by gliding away from the clavicle with the lock and moving the head into side flexion to the opposite side. This can all be highly sensitive so treatment should always be slow.

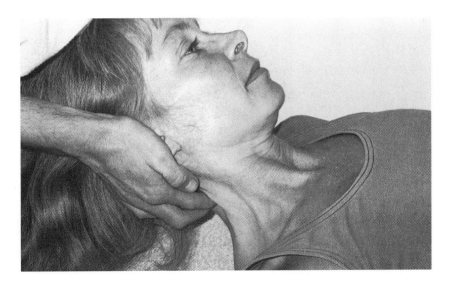

Figure 75: A CTM lock close to the origins of the trapezius as the subject flexes or side flexes the neck.

Neck Extension

Major Muscles: The levator scapulae and splenius cervicis extend the neck. Trapezius, splenius capitis and erector spinae extend the head and the neck. Rectus capitis, posterior major, posterior minor and superior oblique extend the head on the neck.

Neck Rotation

Major Muscles: The semispinalis cervicis, multifidis, scalenus anterior and splenius cervicis rotate the neck. The splenius capitis and SCM rotate the head and the neck. The inferior oblique and the rectus capitis posterior major rotate the head on the neck.

Neck Extensors and Rotators – Treatment

There are two main ways to work this area. Firstly, with the subject in supine position, support his head with one hand and lock with the other as the neck is flexed, side flexed or rotated. The whole of the back and side of the neck must be systematically treated with STR; only minimal movement is required for an effective result. Congestion frequently occurs between the trapezius and the SCM, within the splenius muscles and levator scapulae. These muscles may be reached by locking in deep to the lateral border of the SCM. The trapezius tendons of origin at the occipital need specific attention. Apply a CTM lock as the subject flexes or side flexes his neck to the opposite side (*see* figure 75).

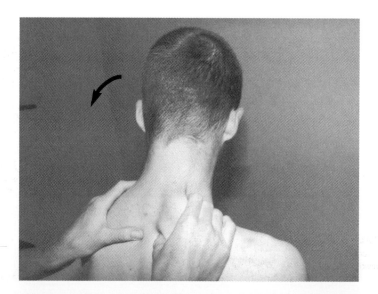

Figure 76: Treatment of the upper fibres of the trapezius with pressure as the neck is flexed or side flexed.

Secondly, in a seated position, the subject can actively move the head as necessary while the therapist locks (*see* figures 71 and 76). It is important to achieve the pressure gently and precisely or movement will be difficult. The trapezius and levator scapulae can be treated highly effectively this way. The insertion point of the levator scapulae can be targeted by curling under the anterior fibres of the trapezius, towards the medial border of the scapula.

Temporomandibular Joint (TMJ)

There are three main muscles associated with this joint; the temporalis, masseter and pterygoids. Problems present as a general aching in the area and/or restricted movement. Dysfunction can occur following a trauma, for example in contact sports or following a whiplash injury. Tissue congestion can develop from a jaw fracture, loss of teeth or after dramatic tooth surgery where the mouth has been forced open for long periods. Chewing on one side of the mouth or clenching the teeth may cause an over-use injury to develop which can lead to pain and headaches.

TMJ – Treatment

Specialist advice may be necessary with problems in this area particularly from a dentist who will check the bite of the subject. STR treatment should consist initially of a general treatment to the neck. To work around the joint, lock in away from the TMJ and instruct the subject to gently open and close his mouth (*see* figure 77). Treatment may help where there is deviation in opening and closing of the jaw.

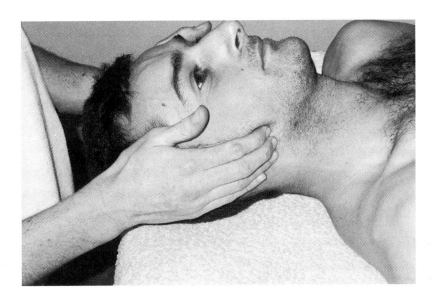

Figure 77: A CTM lock away from the TMJ towards the mouth as the mouth is opened and closed.

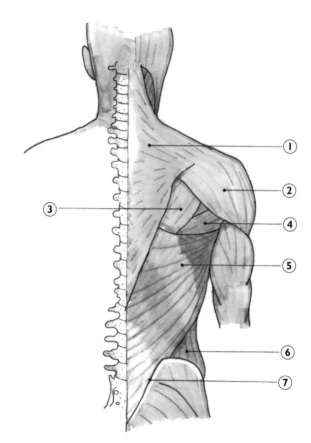

1. Trapezius
2. Posterior deltoid
3. Infraspinatus
4. Teres major
5. Latissimus dorsi
6. External oblique
7. Posterior superior iliac spine
   (PSIS)

Figure 78: Superficial back and shoulder muscles.

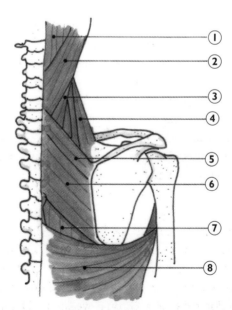

1. Semispinalis capitis
2. Splenius capitis
3. Splenius cervicis
4. Levator scapulae
5. Rhomboid minor
6. Rhomboid major
7. Erector spinae
8. Latissimus dorsi

Figure 79: Deep back and neck muscles.

Part 5
Upper Limb

THE SHOULDER GIRDLE

The scapula is embedded in strong muscles that attach it to the thorax, thoracic spine, neck and head; its only bony connection is to the sternum via the clavicle. This arrangement provides the shoulder girdle with great movement range to facilitate and stabilise immense shoulder mobility.

Muscular imbalance may occur in this area causing postural problems, impaired shoulder movement and pain. Dysfunction in one part of a single muscle can alter the balance of the girdle as a whole, for example, over-use injury to the upper trapezius. Severe shortening and tension in the upper fibres raises the shoulder girdle so that the lower fibres opposing this movement lengthen and become inhibited. A common trunk defect occurring here is that of thoracic kyphosis. In this condition, shoulder girdle protractors tend towards hypertonicity as activities draw the shoulders forward; girdle retractors and trunk extensors become inhibited. Many activities encourage the development of this position, for example working at a computer. Straight back conditions arise as an erect posture is forced and, in this case, it is the retractors and back extensors that become tight and the protractors that become inhibited.

The sternoclavicular and more frequently the acromioclavicular joints can be injured traumatically, particularly in falls. Injury here can lead to future problems with hypermobility, instability and loss of strength. STR around these joints can break adhesive tissue and contribute to healing, reducing the development of a chronic weakness. Maintenance work around the joints to minimise the possibility of an individual developing degenerative conditions from over-use is advantageous for anyone involved with throwing or heavy lifting.

Shoulder Retraction

Major Muscles: Rhomboid major, rhomboid minor and trapezius (middle fibres).

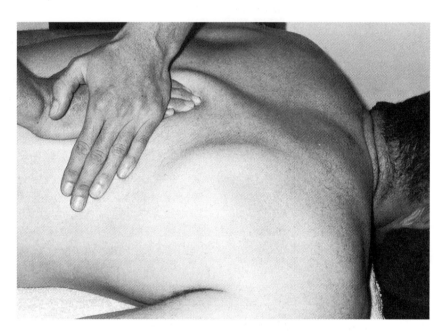

Figure 80: Pressure in the outer border of the lower fibres of the trapezius as the shoulder is elevated.

These muscles work together to produce retraction. The trapezius also assists in lateral rotation, and the rhomboids in medial rotation, of the scapulae. Both muscles are important in stabilising the scapulae during shoulder abduction and adduction. The trapezius has many functions and so plays a crucial role in the overall action of the upper limb.

Shoulder Retractors – Treatment

With the subject in prone position, apply pressure working from the lower to the middle fibres. Lock at points away from the vertebrae, and locate points away from the outer edges of the muscle and its insertion points on the spine of the scapula. Instruct the subject to push his shoulder into the table to produce protraction. As the trapezius is softened, progress to the rhomboids. Providing that there is sufficient flexibility in the muscles and range of movement in the shoulder joint, support the anterior shoulder and move it into medial rotation placing the subject's arm behind his back. This draws the scapula up so that the rhomboid attachments can be easily located along the vertical border (*see* figures 81 and 82). Pressure near to the vertebral attachments must also be administered. After each new lock has been applied, the subject actively protracts by pushing his shoulder into the supporting hand. The rhomboids and trapezius can be targeted effectively from a seated position with passive or active STR (*see* figure 83).

Shoulder Elevation

Major Muscles: Trapezius (upper fibres) and levator scapulae.

As well as elevation the levator scapulae works with the trapezius to produce neck extension when both sides contract. When one side contracts, side flexion occurs. The levator scapulae also assists in medially rotating the scapula.

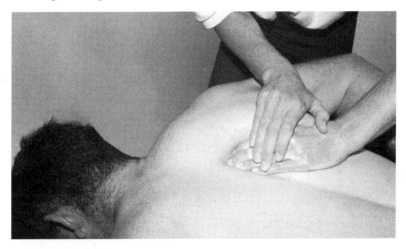

Figure 81: Pressure in the rhomboids as the subject protracts into the table or in this case into the knee of the therapist.

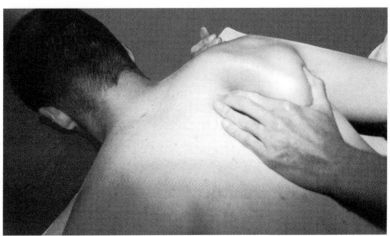

Figure 82: Pressure under the scapula in the rhomboid insertions as the shoulder is protracted into the supporting hand of the therapist.

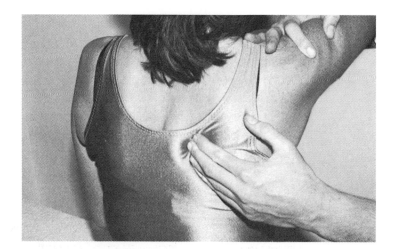

Figure 83: Treatment of the retractors by horizontally adducting the arm to produce shoulder girdle protraction.

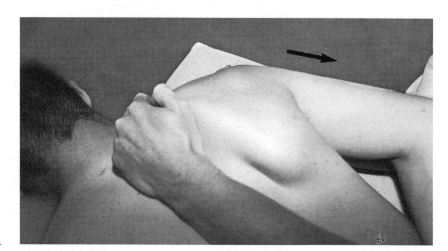

Figure 84: Pressure in the upper fibres of the trapezius as the therapist depresses the shoulder.

Shoulder Elevators – Treatment

With the subject in prone position and supporting his anterior shoulder under one hand, hook over and into the upper fibres of the trapezius with the other. Maintain the lock and depress the shoulder with the supporting hand (*see* figure 84). Working from the head, the trapezius fibres can be targeted as the therapist cups the shoulder with the other hand and pushes it down into depression (*see* figure 85). The levator scapulae may be treated in a similar way; the insertion can be located at the superior angle of the scapula by directing the pressure under the upper trapezius fibres. It may prove easier for the subject to actively depress his shoulder so that the lock can be maintained (*see* figure 86). This will cause considerable release in the area generally.

Shoulder Depression

Major Muscles: Subclavius, pectoralis major, pectoralis minor, trapezius (lower fibres).

The subclavius prevents elevation and protraction of the shoulder girdle.

Shoulder Protraction

Major Muscles: Serratus anterior and pectoralis minor.

The serratus anterior is highly developed in boxers and throwers as punching and throwing require a powerful movement of the scapula forwards. It is important for stabilising the scapula during arm movements and it assists the trapezius in lateral rotation of the scapula. Weakness or

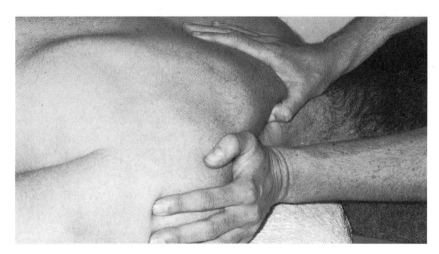

Figure 85: Pressure in the upper fibres of the trapezius as the therapist pushes the shoulder into depression.

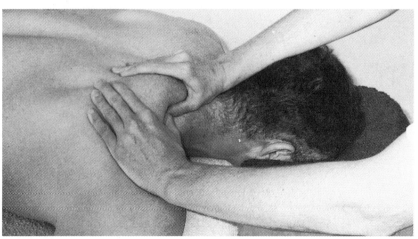

Figure 86: Location of the levator scapulae as the subject depresses his shoulder.

inhibition of this muscle can cause scapula winging. The muscle requires particular attention following dislocation, as it is susceptible to strength loss. The pectoralis minor assists the serratus anterior in protraction and also raises the ribs to assist in forced inspiration.

Shoulder Protractors – Treatment

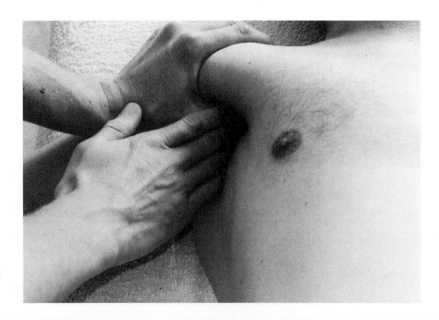

1. Subclavius
2. Coracobrachialis
3. Subscapularis
4. Pectoralis minor
5. Serratus anterior
6. Biceps brachii

Figure 87: Chest and anterior shoulder – deep muscles.

With the subject in supine position, the pectoralis minor can be reached specifically by abducting the arm to 90 degrees and gently delving under the pectoralis major, towards the coracoid process and the origin of the muscle. Once reached, the depth should be maintained whilst the subject raises his arm to draw the scapula upwards. Alternatively, a movement of retraction can occur if he pushes his posterior shoulder or arm down into the table. Either way, the pressure needs to be released promptly (*see* figure 88). STR to the serratus anterior is most easily administered with the subject in side lying position. The muscle may be targeted as the arm is extended to produce retraction of the shoulder girdle (*see* figure 89).

Figure 88: Pressure towards the pectoralis minor as the subject raises his arm.

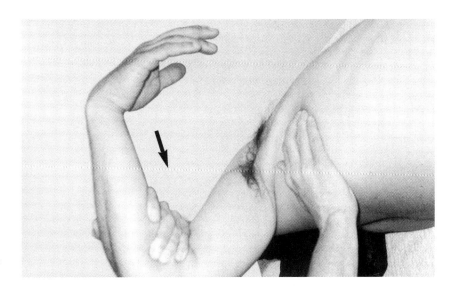

Figure 89: Pressure in the serratus anterior as the girdle is retracted.

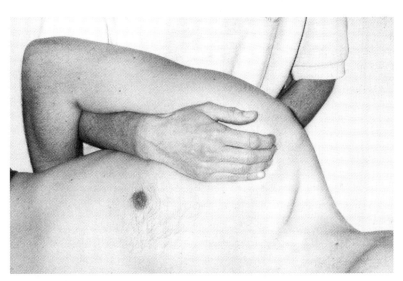

Figure 90: Treatment of the trapezius in a side lying position, anterior view.

Shoulder Girdle in Side Lying and Seated Positions – Treatment

With the subject side lying and his arm behind him, secure his anterior shoulder and use both hands to move the scapula. It is important not to force this position if the subject has any restriction; treatment should continue by allowing his arm to relax in front. Once in position, focused locks and small precise active movements of retraction, protraction, elevation and depression alongside appropriate locks may be highly effective in freeing the girdle as a whole. Scapula movement, or lack of, can be assessed well in this position so treatment can have rapid results (*see* figures 90 and 91).

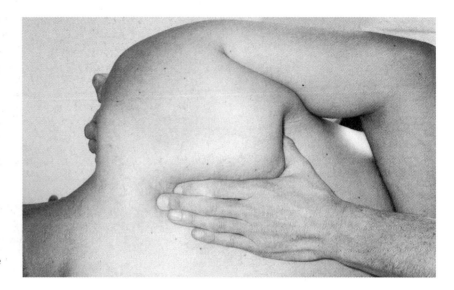

Figure 91: Treatment of the shoulder girdle muscles in a side lying position, posterior view.

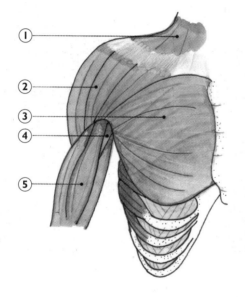

1. Platysma
2. Anterior deltoid
3. Pectoralis major
4. Coracobrachialis
5. Biceps brachii

Figure 92: Chest and anterior shoulder.

With the subject seated, active STR can be administered easily into the trapezius and rhomboids as the subject protracts by pushing his shoulder forward. A resistance can be given here to enhance the release. The lower fibres can be located as the subject elevates the girdle by shrugging his shoulders. Very dynamic active STR can be conducted using broad active arm movements to produce the required shoulder girdle action (*see* figure 83).

THE SHOULDER

The structure of the shoulder joint allows for an excellent range of movement, but because of this, it lacks passive stability and has to rely heavily on the strength of its surrounding muscles. Any muscular dysfunction, therefore, will affect the strength of the joint itself. Following injury, STR within all movements is necessary so that an imbalance or restriction does not affect shoulder mobility and strength.

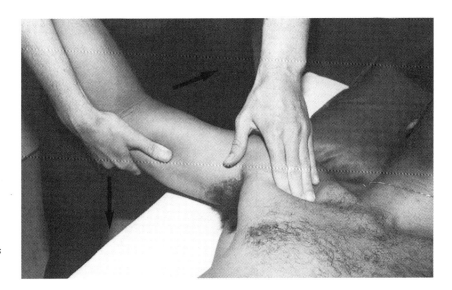

Figure 93: Pressure in the clavicular fibres of the pectoralis major as the therapist abducts the arm.

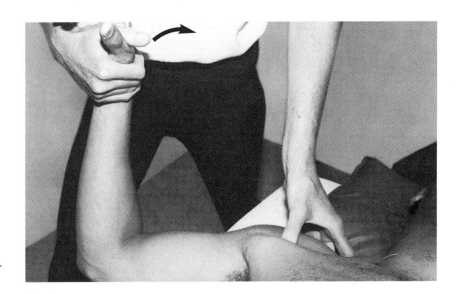

Figure 94: Pressure in the anterior deltoid as the shoulder is laterally rotated.

Shoulder Flexion

Major Muscles: Pectoralis major (clavicular fibres), anterior deltoid, long head of biceps brachii, coracobrachialis.

The pectoralis major works in conjunction with the anterior deltoid and the protractors by moving the arm forwards in pushing, punching and throwing movements. It is also strong in adduction, particularly in the horizontal plane.

Shoulder Flexors – Treatment

In supine position, secure the subject's arm by grasping the elbow, to ensure his relaxation. Treat the pectoralis major by locking in at points off the sternum and the clavicle and conduct combination movements of shoulder extension and abduction to produce a stretch (*see* figure 93). Progress to treating the whole muscle. Towards the insertion points, angle the lock carefully as the anterior shoulder is a sensitive area. Taking hold of the subject's hand and producing a lateral rotation movement here provides a highly effective stretch that also works well for the anterior deltoid (*see* figure 94). The long head of the biceps and the coracobrachialis can be treated by first shortening the muscle, locking and extending the shoulder. Precise locks delving between seemingly 'stringy' tendons will provide a noticeable release in this sensitive area.

Shoulder Extension

Major Muscles: Latissimus dorsi, teres major, posterior deltoid and the long head of triceps brachii.

Shoulder Adduction

Major Muscles: Latissimus dorsi, teres major, pectoralis major and coracobrachialis.

The latissimus dorsi is the widest muscle of the back and is a powerful adductor and extensor of the shoulder. With the arms fixed above the

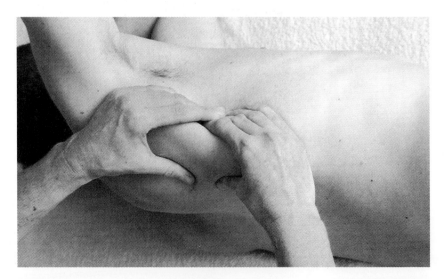

Figure 95: Pressure in the latissimus dorsi as the shoulder is flexed or abducted.

head, it draws the body up together with the pectoralis major, for example in the performance of chin-ups and dips, in the down stroke of the front crawl swimming cycle and in climbing. Strains can occur at the tendon insertion, where tiny STR stretching movements incorporating rotation are beneficial. The teres major, often termed as the 'little helper' to the latissimus dorsi, assists these muscles but is only effective if the scapula is fixed, by the rhomboids. All three muscles are important for shoulder stability.

Shoulder Extensors and Adductors – Treatment

With the subject prone, lock at points along the latissimus dorsi up until its insertion at the humerus. For the teres major, treat from the origin at the inferior angle of the scapula and apply pressure at points along the muscle to its insertion point. Each time, lock and take the shoulder into abduction. This can also be done side lying where it is easier to instruct the subject into active and resisted movements (*see* figures 95 and 96). If the therapist hooks under the latissimus dorsi, away from the serratus anterior, an active flexion movement will provide a significant stretch to the muscle and fascia. The posterior deltoid and long head of the triceps brachii can also be treated with flexion movements.

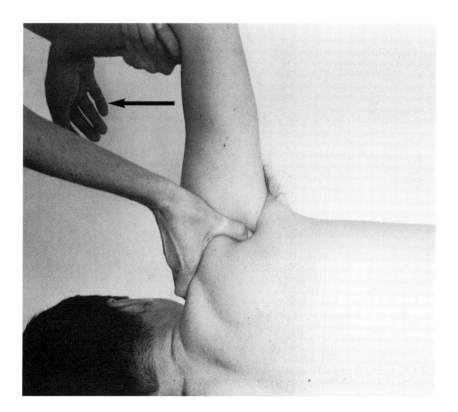

Figure 96: Treatment of the teres major in the side lying position by locking and abducting or laterally rotating the shoulder.

Shoulder Abduction

Major Muscles: Medial deltoid and supraspinatus.

Any movement of the humerus in the scapula will involve the deltoids. The supraspinatus assists the medial deltoid in shoulder abduction.

Shoulder Abductors – Treatment

Good results can be obtained with the subject seated upright. In the anterior deltoid, the lock is enforced while the shoulder is actively extended; in the posterior deltoid, it is enforced while the shoulder is flexed. The medial fibres can be shortened slightly and locked into as the arm is adducted, but this is difficult particularly on strong deltoids. Alternatively these muscles may be treated with the subject side lying where active shoulder rotation may also be incorporated to stretch the fibres. Rotation should be lateral to stretch the anterior fibres and medial to stretch the posterior fibres (*see* figure 97). The medial deltoid fibres can be locked into while the subject pushes into his side and this will provide a subtle STR effect.

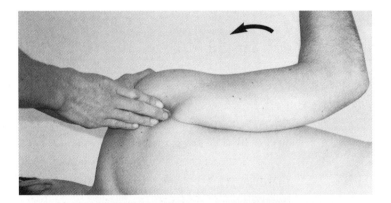

Figure 97: Pressure in the posterior deltoid as the subject medially rotates the arm.

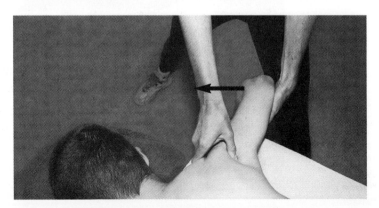

Figure 98: Pressure in the teres major as the therapist moves the arm into lateral rotation or abduction.

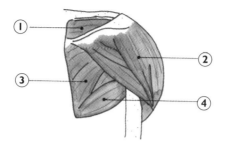

1. Supraspinatus
2. Posterior deltoid
3. Infraspinatus
4. Teres major

Figure 99: Posterior shoulder.

For treatment of the supraspinatus, position the subject prone with his shoulder slightly abducted. Prior to administering STR to this muscle, ensure that the upper trapezius has been sufficiently relaxed; then apply a deep pressure into the supraspinatus by hooking the fingers into the fossa area as the subject adducts the shoulder slowly. Follow this by applying CTM locks at points away from the spine of the scapula, superior to it, each time guiding the subject into shoulder adduction (*see* also page 93).

Lateral Rotation

Major Muscles: Teres minor, infraspinatus and posterior deltoid.

Medial Rotation

Major Muscles: Subscapularis, teres major, latissimus dorsi, pectoralis major and anterior deltoid.

Rotator Cuff Muscles

The Muscles: Subscapularis, supraspinatus, infraspinatus and teres minor.

These muscles are essential for keeping the head of the humerus in the glenoid fossa during arm movement. They also inhibit upward displacement of the head when the biceps, triceps and deltoids are active. They are vulnerable to over-use and traumatic injury. Loss of a particular rotation is a common symptom in shoulder pain. As the rotator cuff works collectively, the massage therapist should work on all these muscles to encourage rebalance as well as the other muscles involved with rotation such as the posterior deltoid and latissimus dorsi. To test for rotation, ask the subject to put his palmar hand on the back of his head for lateral rotation; to test for medial rotation, ask him to place his dorsal hand on the small of his back.

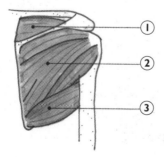

1. Supraspinatus
2. Infraspinatus
3. Teres major

Figure 100: Posterior shoulder – deep muscles.

Shoulder Problems

With any dysfunction or reduced range of movement in this area, it is imperative to address the shoulder girdle musculature, in particular the serratus anterior, pectoralis minor and upper fibres of the trapezius towards the acromion.

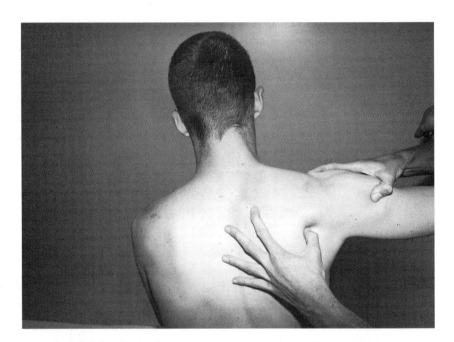

Figure 101: Treatment of the infraspinatus in a seated position by locking and medially rotating the shoulder.

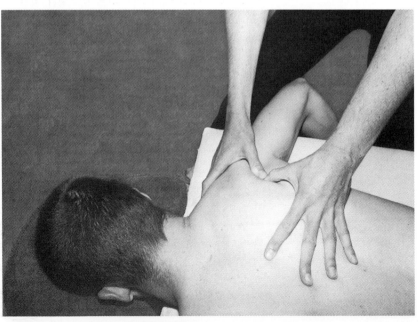

Figure 102: Pressure in the infraspinatus as the subject moves into medial rotation.

Impingement syndrome refers to the pain and pressure exerted on the rotator cuff tendons, positioned under the coracoacromial arch, during shoulder elevation. The impingement can be caused by 'overcrowding' of the subacromial space and by weakness and imbalance of the rotator cuff. STR applied to the shoulder girdle and rotator cuff muscles is extremely beneficial in the early stages of these injuries, but it is essential that the underlying causes of the injury are addressed.

Careful treatment of the muscles will alleviate tendinitis. The supraspinatus tendon (supraspinatus tendinitis) and the long head of the biceps tendon are the most commonly affected.

'Frozen shoulder' ultimately refers to capsulitis of the shoulder joint which severely reduces rotation and abduction. Addressing the rotator cuff muscles, in particular the subscapularis, can have positive results on this very painful condition. As controlled movement is a positive step for all healing, gentle STR can work well in alleviating discomfort and speeding the healing processes.

Rotator Cuff – Treatment

With the subject in prone position, apply CTM locks at points on the scapula, the infraspinatus and teres minor, and perform passive STR by slowly taking the shoulder into medial rotation. Once the area is warmed up, instruct him into an active movement of medial rotation (*see* figure 102). Progress to the supraspinatus. Given that the upper fibres of the trapezius have been softened, gently apply a deep pressure into the muscle

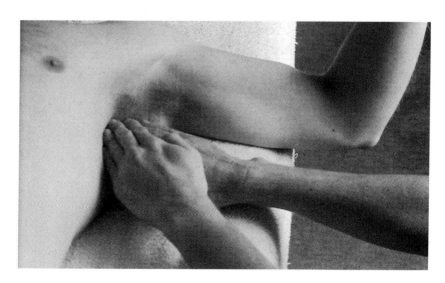

Figure 103: Pressure towards the subscapularis as the subject laterally rotates the shoulder.

and direct active adduction of the shoulder. The musculotendinous junction can be treated with the arm supported and abducted to 90 degrees. The actual insertion can be easily located by medially rotating the arm to make the attachment point more forward and superficial. In both these positions, it is possible to lock as the subject produces a movement; resisted STR may prove useful. The subscapularis is best treated in supine position with the arm abducted to 90 degrees. Lock onto the anterior surface of the scapula and slowly laterally rotate the shoulder (*see* figure 103). All this can be a tough and sensitive area to work so each point should not be laboured; rather the whole area should be covered systematically. Active STR is extremely useful as re-education is occurring; also it ensures movement within the subject's range and not beyond.

THE ELBOW

Joint stability at the elbow, is predominantly provided by the collateral ligaments and musculature around the elbow. The neck should be considered during treatment of any over-use injury to the elbow. Inflammation on the lateral and medial elbow are related to the muscles producing wrist movements. Common over-use problems originate in faulty technique and repetitive gripping and extension of the elbow such as in racquet sports.

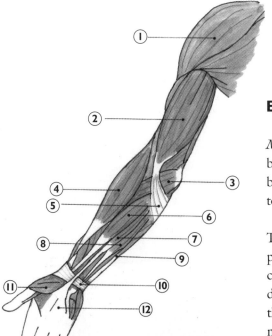

1. Anterior deltoid
2. Biceps brachii
3. Pronator teres
4. Brachioradialis
5. Bicipital aponeurosis
6. Flexor carpi radialis
7. Palmaris longus
8. Flexor digitorum
   superficialis
9. Flexor carpi ulnaris
10. Flexor retinaculum
11. Thenar eminence
12. Palmar aponeurosis

Figure 104: Anterior arm – superficial muscles.

Elbow Flexion

Major Muscles: Biceps brachii, brachialis, brachioradialis, pronator teres.

The brachialis is the primary elbow flexor and controls the movement during extension. It has the capacity to develop myositis ossificans so extreme care should be taken following a direct trauma. The biceps brachii is a strong supinator as well as an elbow flexor and these actions are often performed together. The muscle also contributes to shoulder flexion and stability of the joint. It is the long head that is more prone to injury. The brachioradialis as a flexor works strongly when the elbow is midway between either pronation or supination.

Elbow Extension

Major Muscles: Triceps brachii and anconeus.

The triceps are the only muscle on the posterior of the upper arm. Because the triceps work strongly in fast elbow extension movements, they are exercised in any pushing movements, for example dips and push-ups. Punching or throwing can stress the attachments. Actual strains are rare but bad technique can cause pain and tearing particularly at the musculotendinous junction. The anconeus controls extension movements.

Pronation of Forearm

Major Muscles: Pronator teres, pronator quadratus and brachioradialis.

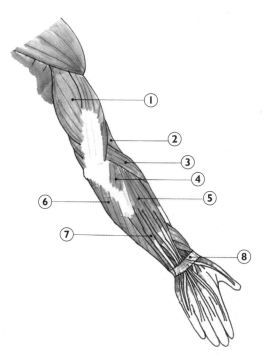

The pronator teres works strongly alongside the flexors during pronation and flexion movements such as the grip in horse riding. The pronator quadratus is stronger if the pronation is conducted with the elbow extension.

1. Triceps
2. Brachioradialis
3. Extensor carpi radialis longus
4. Anconeus
5. Extensor digitorum
6. Flexor carpi ulnaris
7. Extensor carpi ulnaris
8. Extensor retinaculum

Figure 105: Posterior arm – superficial muscles.

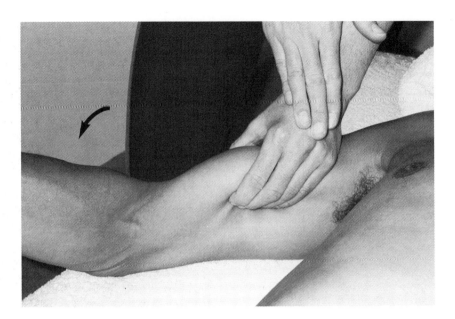

Figure 106: Pressure on either side of the biceps brachii as the elbow is extended.

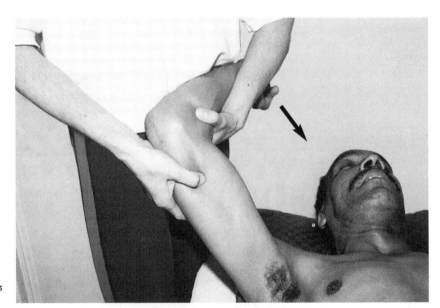

Figure 107: Pressure in the triceps brachii as the elbow is flexed.

Supination of Forearm

Major Muscles: Supinator, biceps brachii and brachioradialis.

The biceps brachii is the strongest muscle in supination. The supinator is exercised most strongly if combined with elbow extension and has sufficient strength for slow movements with minimal resistance.

Elbow – Treatment

With the subject supine and the elbow flexed, gently grasp either side of the belly of the biceps. Extend and pronate to stretch (*see* figure 106). Treat the whole muscle paying particular attention to the origins carefully angling the locks due to the sensitivity of the area. Treat the lateral side and direct the lock under the biceps to work the brachialis. With the shoulder fully flexed by the subject's ear, lock into points along the triceps and flex the elbow (*see* figure 107). Pay close attention to the tendon attachments. The supinators and pronators in the forearm can be worked well by incorporating combination movements of supination, pronation with flexion and extension of the wrist to separate the forearm as a whole.

THE WRIST

As with the ankle, there is a band of connective tissue that supports the many tendons that attach across the wrist joint. The space created underneath the flexor retinaculum is known as the carpal tunnel. The flexor pollicis longus, flexor digitorum profundus and flexor digitorum superficialis as well as the median nerve all pass through this 'tunnel'. The posterior retinaculum makes six compartments for the extensor tendons.

Carpal tunnel syndrome is a result of congestion in the tunnel. Any repetitive actions involving the flexors, such as gripping, can cause inflammation in the tendons. If numbness and tingling are present then the median nerve is also affected. STR works well to separate the tendons and

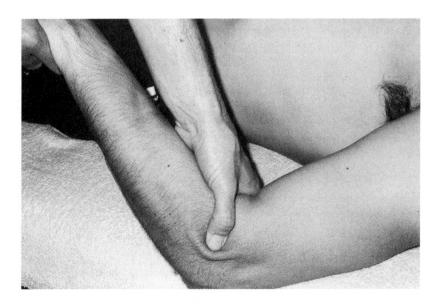

Figure 108: Pressure in the common extensor origin of the elbow as the wrist is flexed.

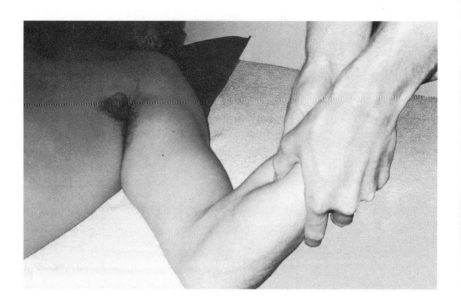

Figure 109: Pressure in the forearm flexors as the wrist is extended.

adhesions between them and the retinaculum. Frequently this condition is corrected successfully by surgery but the use of STR at an early stage can make this unnecessary.

Repetitive strain injury (RSI) occurs with over-use and subsequent adherence and inflammation of the tendons in the posterior compartment. Activities such as typing or playing the piano repetitively, or racquet sports where the extensors contract eccentrically to brace and control the force during backhand shots, can all cause degrees of RSI.

Wrist sprains are common in contact sports and STR is a good form of early treatment to ensure good strength gains. With any wrist problem a systematic treatment of the whole forearm and hand is necessary. Abduction, adduction, flexion and extension need to be considered. At the wrist, STR can separate adherence between the individual tendons and the retinaculum.

Wrist Extension

Major Muscles: Extensor carpi radialis longus, extensor carpi radialis brevis, extensor carpi ulnaris, extensor digitorum communis, extensor indicis, extensor digiti minimi, extensor pollicis longus and extensor pollicis brevis.

Pain occurring at the lateral side of the elbow is often classified under the umbrella term of 'tennis elbow', or lateral epicondylitis. There are many different origins of this pain including nerve entrapment, bursitis and tendinitis. Commonly the term refers to over-use leading to injury and inflammation of the common extensor origin (CEO) resulting in fibrous tissue in the tendon, musculotendinous junction, or at the tenoperiosteal junction. In conjunction with RICE and stretching, STR is an invaluable tool in the management of tennis elbow. A general forearm massage should be conducted prior to focusing on the adhesive tissue.

Wrist Flexion

Major Muscles: Flexor carpi ulnaris, flexor carpi radialis, palmaris longus, flexor digitorum superficialis, flexor digitorum profundus and flexor pollicis longus.

Pain on the medial elbow is generalised as 'golfer's elbow' or medial epicondylitis, where inflammation develops at the common flexor origin (CFO). It is less common than lateral elbow pain and usually responds to treatment faster.

Wrist Abduction

Major Muscles: Flexor carpi radialis, extensor carpi radialis longus, extensor carpi radialis brevis, abductor pollicis longus and extensor pollicis brevis jointly produce wrist abduction (radial deviation).

Wrist Adduction

Major Muscles: Flexor carpi ulnaris and extensor carpi ulnaris work together in wrist adduction (ulna deviation).

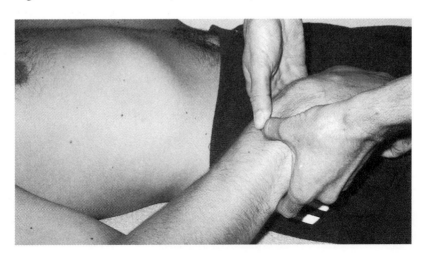

Figure 110: Pressure between the extensor tendons as the wrist is flexed.

Wrist – Treatment

With the subject in supine position, apply STR to the extensors from the wrist to the elbow by locking in and flexing the wrist. Concentrate on locking between the extensor muscles to stretch the fascia where congestion and adherence are often present. If there is any form of 'tennis elbow' progress to the tendinous attachment (CEO) and apply a CTM lock as the subject flexes his wrist (*see* figure 108). Locate points at the back of the wrist separating the extensor tendons from the retinaculum. Avoid irritating areas of inflammation, and instead, concentrate on releasing the congestion around it.

Treat the flexors in the same manner but lock and extend the wrist to release the tension (*see* figure 109). Applying pressure between the flexor tendons at the wrist will relieve carpal tunnel syndrome; this release may be enhanced by incorporating either abduction or adduction following the wrist flexion.

THE HAND

The thenar eminence is formed by the flexor pollicis brevis, the abductor pollicis brevis and the opponens pollicis. The hypothenar eminence is formed by the flexor digiti minimi, the abductor digiti minimi and the opponens digiti minimi. The 'anatomical snuffbox' is a depression in the dorsum of the first metacarpal with the extensor pollicis brevis forming its lateral border and the extensor pollicis longus forming its medial border. De Quervain's syndrome is tenovaginitis or tenosynovitis affecting the extensor pollicis brevis and the abductor pollicis longus.

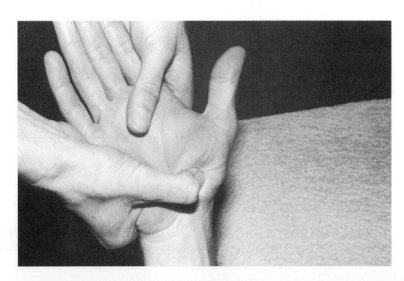

Figure 111: Pressure in the thenar eminence as the thumb is extended.

Finger Flexion

Major Muscles: Flexor digitorum superficialis, flexor digitorum profundus, lumbricals, interossei and flexor digiti minimi brevis.

Finger Extension

Major Muscles: Extensor digitorum communis, extensor digiti minimi, extensor indicis, interossei, lumbricals.

Thumb Flexion

Major Muscles: Flexor pollicis longus, opponens pollicis and flexor pollicis brevis.

Thumb Extension

Major Muscles: Extensor pollicis longus, extensor pollicis brevis and abductor pollicis longus.

Thumb Abduction

Major Muscles: Abductor pollicis longus and abductor pollicis brevis.

Thumb Adduction

Major Muscle: Adductor pollicis.

Opposing Thumb

Major Muscles: Opponens pollicis and flexor pollicis brevis.

Lumbricals and Interossei

Flexion of metacarpo-phalangeal joints with simultaneous extension of interphalangeal joints.

Finger Abduction

Major Muscles: Dorsal interossei, abductor digiti minimi and abductor pollicis brevis.

Finger Adduction

Major Muscles: Palmar interossei and adductor pollicis.

Opposing Fingers

Major Muscle: Opponens digiti minimi.

The Hand – Treatment

Sprained fingers and thumbs are injuries especially common in ball sports and gymnastics. STR will speed the recovery of healing. For the thenar eminence, lock while the subject straightens the thumb in all directions (*see* figure 111). For the hypothenar eminence, lock and straighten the little finger. Treat the extensors over the top of the hand by locking across and in between them and flexing the metacarpals; the finger extensors should be considered in conjunction with the forearm extensors and the palmar hand together with the wrist flexors.

Part 6

Pre- and Post-event Treatment

EVENT MASSAGE

Event massage means treating an athlete with a particular performance in mind. It can both enhance performance and speed up the recovery processes afterwards. Many 'elite' sports people recognise this now and have their own massage therapists who travel with them. Recognition of the value of such treatment is also beginning to infiltrate at club level sports and dance, so the demand for sports massage therapy at events is increasing rapidly.

Pre-event Massage

Pre-event massage may be conducted days before an event; general massage before an event will ensure that the body is functioning freely and that the athlete maintains the physical condition that is essential if he is to 'peak' at the all-important time. Sometimes a particular area is causing concern and the therapist can use STR to pinpoint and concentrate on this area. Deep, preventative massage can be conducted up to about two days before an event, according to client preference; a much more gentle approach must be taken any closer to the event because soreness often follows a deep treatment.

Many sports people in the competitive arena would prefer not to have treatment very close to their event if they find that the therapy involved is not conducive to the mental state they require for their event. This may be, for example, if they find treatment very relaxing at a time when they are trying to develop a mood of aggression so that they can perform to their maximum. There are, of course, no hard and fast rules for this as each individual is different. Obviously it is better if the athlete and therapist have already worked together so that the therapist understands the mental outlook and individual preferences of the athlete as well as the physical aspects involved. Then athlete and therapist can work in partnership towards the actual event in mutual understanding and trust. If you do not know the athlete well, you must be aware that psychological as well as physical preparation is important and so you should respect his decision about how soon before the event the treatment should be given.

Pre Warm-up Massage

It is becoming increasingly common for pre-event massage to take place at the sports venue prior to the event but then its exact nature will vary widely according to the subject. An experienced athlete who has trained for an event invariably knows exactly how he wants to feel, physically and mentally, to perform well; this is not only because of individual character differences but also because of the demands of the particular event. Some events require the athlete to be keyed up like a coiled spring ready to bound into action as may be the case prior to explosive type events such as weight lifting. Others, such as archery or shooting, require a relaxed and calm approach. Thus, some athletes may choose not to have treatment immediately prior to warm-up while others might be keen to have it. The type of treatment will depend, therefore, both on individual preference and the nature of the event.

After Warm-up or as Part of the Warm-up Massage

Given the constraints and drawbacks of conventional massage immediately prior to performance, STR has several advantages to offer. For one thing, it can be done actively. Most competitions require a high degree of physical activity in which case warm-up procedures involve a progression to dynamic movement. Whereas a relaxing massage using deep, slow effleurage and kneading could be mentally wrong and physically make an athlete feel lethargic, weak or too relaxed, STR can be done very dynamically. The therapist can use active functional work where the athlete is producing the actual movement so that he still feels in control of the preparation and warm-up. This removes the disadvantage of massage being

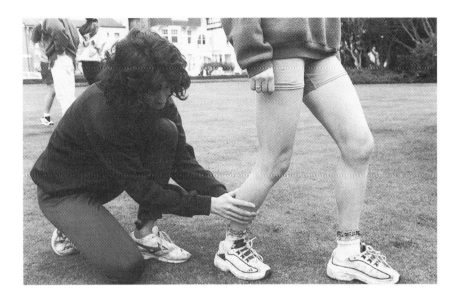

Figure 112: A pre-event treatment on the calf muscles with STR in a weight-bearing position.

too mentally relaxing. Another advantage of STR where treatment is being given at an actual meet, is its versatility. It is so easy to improvise when there is no treatment couch. Work can quite easily be done sitting, kneeling, or on the floor and this informality mixes well with the mounting excitement that is part of the mental preparation. STR can be conducted with the athlete standing and weight bearing, for example with the calves. It can also be administered through clothes without using oil or lotion; this has obvious benefits particularly in cold weather when no shelter is available. Yet another advantage of STR in a pre-event situation is its economy of time. In team sports it would be impossible to give everyone in the squad a general pre-event massage if you were the only therapist. With the use of STR, attention can be given to all team members, if necessary, as key areas can be treated quickly and precisely without any time wastage.

Pre-event Massage and Injury

As an event approaches, an athlete may suffer from a particular injury and be faced with the difficult decision of whether or not to compete. For someone at the pinnacle of a career, it is difficult to turn down an exciting opportunity and so a decision is made to risk further injury or a disappointing performance and compete anyway. Ultimately it is a very personal decision and the therapist, though able to advise, is bound to accept it. In this case, the aim of treatment is not to 'cure' but to enable the athlete to compete more comfortably with less risk of worsening the injury; the therapist must help the athlete to manage and alleviate the symptoms. Exactly which treatment is given will depend on how imminent the event is. True healing needs time to work as it involves biological processes. In many cases the body can react to initial treatment negatively, as the breakage of scarring and separation of adhesion can leave residual discomfort or inflammation. By definition, time is exactly what is not available at a pre-event treatment.

If administering to an injury prior to an event, it should be made clear to the athlete that the treatment is not a cure but only an interim measure to help alleviate symptoms. Then a controlled approach, rather than a treatment approach is adopted. Here is an example:

A middle distance runner is competing at a top-level competition where he is expected to reach the final but a bad shin splint type of condition presents itself. The cure for this condition would probably be a course of treatment involving deep work close to the shin breaking adhesions but each of these treatments would leave the runner feeling initially sore, bruised and unable to run well. In this case, as an interim measure, careful usage of STR could take some of the stress away from the injury, so alleviating the pain though not actually removing the cause. In conjunction with periodic icing, gentle treatment to the whole lower leg around the adhesive tissue would ensure maximal release and minimal aggravation so giving the athlete a chance of running as well as he would without the injury. More work should be conducted in and after the warm-down and the athlete should be made aware of what needs to be done for an actual cure.

In brief, pre-event massage for injury involves the control approach: it should be non-invasive and non-aggravating with the aim of decongesting and aiding movement and function where possible. It can be used in conjunction with ice. The subject must understand the limitations of what is being done.

Post-event Massage

The main objectives of post-event massage are to speed up the subject's recovery time and to ensure maximum return to full function. It should not be seen as an alternative to warm-down procedures though, if an athlete is so exhausted or injured that warm-down exercise is impossible, post-event massage will be a good compensation; this is because, like warm-down, it removes muscle waste by enhancing circulation and it stretches the tissues.

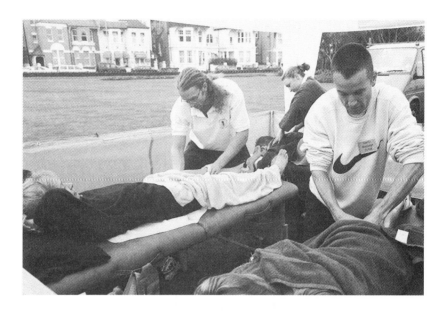

Figure 113: Runners enjoying a post-event massage following the Hastings half marathon.

As well as giving both mental and physical relaxation, post-race massage helps lessen the possibility of injury and enables the athlete to get back to training more quickly than would otherwise be the case.

It is important that the subject should understand that post-race massage is not curative. Immediately after an event, when an athlete is perhaps exhausted, dehydrated, and susceptible to cramp, is not the right time to delve into adhesion and inflammation. Instead, muscles need to be gently relieved of their congestion by elongating and stretching fibres. The

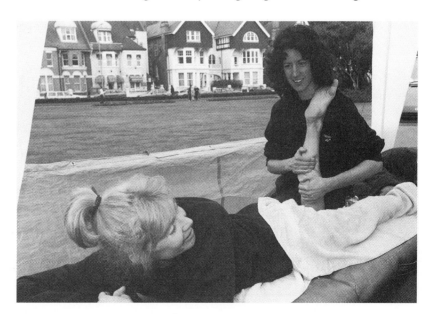

Figure 114: Post-event massage should be gentle consisting primarily of traditional massage strokes: effleurage and kneading.

therapist applies soothing and recuperative massage that makes the muscles pliant and soft. If there is an actual 'injury', it is better simply to apply ice, leaving specific treatment until after recuperation from the event. Usage of STR may be minimal or very gentle; effleurage and kneading strokes should dominate the post-event massage.

As with pre-event massage, improvisation, versatility and expertise are needed to cope with post-event massage because unpredictable factors invariably arise. For example weather conditions may bring about added difficulties and time management is almost bound to be difficult: sometimes the therapist may be trying to cope with a queue of cold athletes with very little shelter available. It is all a part of the challenge of event massage!

Between Event Massage

Occasionally the therapist is asked to help someone in a situation that is a combination of pre- and post-event. Examples of this include; between scenes at a dance performance; a decathlon competition; between an individual race and a team relay. In such cases, a combination of recovery and preparatory techniques is required. Obviously the therapist will need to use judgement and experience to assess physical factors and will also need to be extremely sensitive to the mental state of the subject.

Event massage can be extremely exciting and rewarding; it can also be emotionally draining as the therapist shares the athlete's hopes, anxieties and anticipations. Ultimately, it is one of the most rewarding aspects of sports massage.

Part 7
Self-treatment

Correct usage of self-treatment will aid the recovery of tension from hard training or from a tough day at the office! Often a therapist is not available or lack of time or money make it impossible to have regular treatment. Frequent short sessions of self-treatment can make a huge difference in minimising the risk of injury.

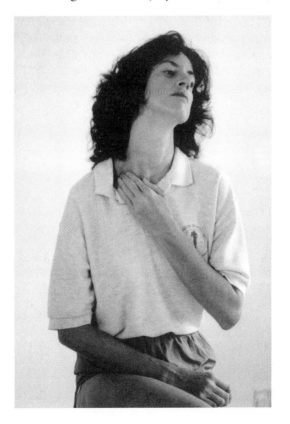

Figure 115: A CTM lock as the head is extended and rotated.

STR is easier to administer on yourself than many massage techniques because the muscles do not have to be totally relaxed for treatment to take place. Also, because much of the technique is active, all the subject has to do is locate the problem area and move into a stretch. The dynamic nature of STR makes it simple to deliver to yourself.

In fact, it is almost instinctive. If someone has a stiff neck you may see them clutching at

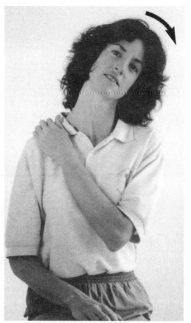

their upper trapezius and moving their head from side to side or shrugging their shoulder. A little guidance would actually make this quite effective at relieving the adherence and hypertonicity.

Self-treatment is also a must for any therapist who is at risk of developing over-use injuries in his elbows wrists and thumbs. These areas are easy to reach so maintenance should be easy!

The following are a few examples but they are by no means exhaustive. Before long the therapist will be able to treat his own psoas without any worries!

Figure 116: Pressure in the upper trapezius as the head is side flexed.

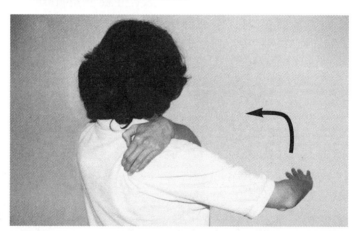

Figure 117: Pressure in the trapezius as the arm is moved to protract the shoulder girdle.

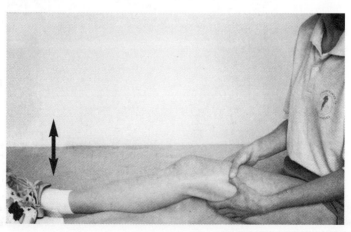

Figure 118: Pressure in the quadriceps as the knee is flexed from a straight leg position.

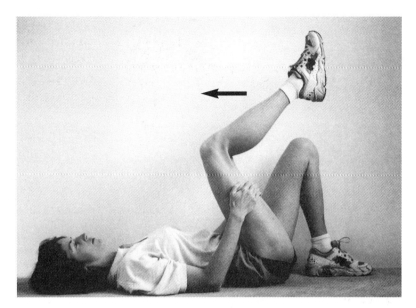

Figure 119: Locking into the hamstrings as the leg is straightened for a stretch.

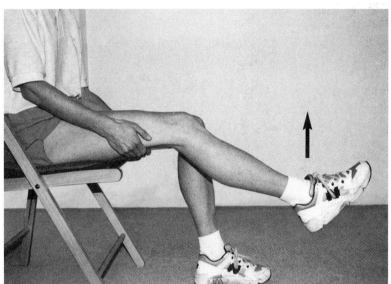

Figure 120: Pressure in the hamstrings as a stretch is produced from a seated position.

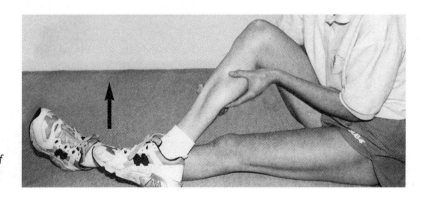

Figure 121: Locking into the calf to provide valuable relief, as the foot is dorsiflexed.

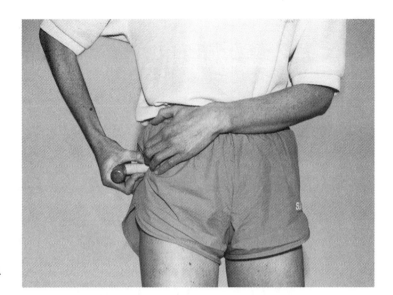

Figure 122: The use of a wooden peg to lock into the TFL as the hip is moved laterally.

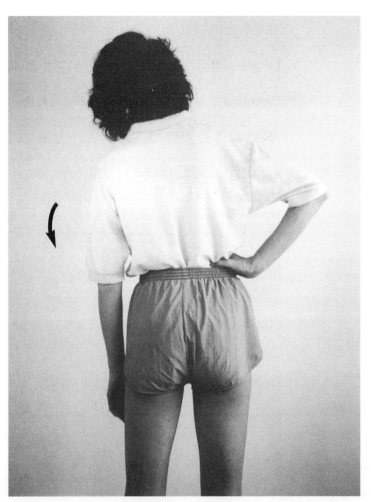

Figure 123: Pressure towards the quadratus lumborum as the spine is side flexed.

Appendix 1
Anatomical Movements

Flexion	Reduction in joint angle during movement.
Extension	Increase in joint angle during movement.
Abduction	Movement away from the midline of the body.
Adduction	Movement towards the midline of the body.
Medial Rotation	Rotation around a longitudinal axis towards the midline of the body.
Lateral Rotation	Rotation around a longitudinal axis away from the midline of the body.
Circumduction	Combination of flexion, extension, abduction, adduction, medial and lateral rotation.
Elevation	Movement upwards.
Depression	Movement downwards.
Retraction	Movement of the scapulae backwards towards the midline of the body.

Protraction	Movement of the scapulae forwards.
Lateral Rotation of the Scapula	Movement of the inferior angle of the scapula laterally as the acromion moves into elevation.
Medial Rotation of the Scapula	Return of the inferior angle medially as the acromion moves into depression.
Supination	Movement of the palm face upwards.
Pronation	Movement of the palm face downwards.
Plantar Flexion	Movement of the sole of the foot downwards.
Dorsiflexion	Movement of the top of the foot to the anterior of the tibia.
Eversion	Turning of the sole outward so that the weight is on the inside edge of the foot.
Inversion	Turning of the sole inward so that the weight is on the outside edge of the foot.
Toe Flexion	Movement of the toes to the floor.
Toe Extension	Movement of the toes upward.

Appendix 2
Common Postural Deficiencies

SIDE VIEW

Head Position   Excessive inward curve (convex) of the cervical spine, poking the chin forwards.

Thoracic Kyphosis   Exaggerated concave curve of the thoracic spine.

Straight Back   Reduction in the concave curve of the thoracic spine.

Lumbar Lordosis   Excessive convex curve of the lumbar spine.

Flat Back   Reduction of the convex curve of the lumbar spine.

Pelvic Position   Anterior or posterior tilt of the pelvis.

Sway Back   The pelvis is positioned forwards, in either a neutral or posteriorly tilted position, in relation to the back and legs.

Genu Recurvatum   Sway-back knees.

Pes Planus and Pes Cavus   Flat foot and high arch.

POSTERIOR VIEW

Head Position	Head turned to one side.
Scoliosis	Lateral deviation or curve of the spine.
Scapulae Positions	Level of inferior angles of scapulae. Level of acromion processes. Scapulae winging.
PSIS Positions	Level of posterior superior iliac spines.
Genu Valgum and Genu Varum	Knock-knee and bow-leg.
Foot Position	Excessive eversion (pronation) of the mid-foot, calcaneal eversion or inversion.

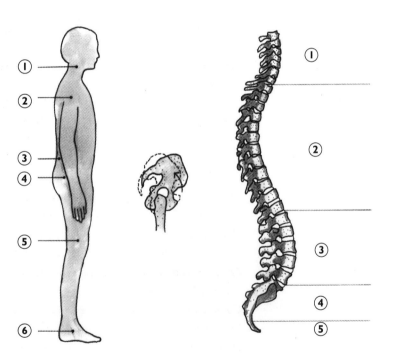

1. Neck
2. Shoulder girdle
3. Lumbar
4. Pelvis
5. Knees
6. Feet

Figure 124: Postural balance.

1. Cervical curve
2. Thoracic curve
3. Lumbar curve
4. Sacrum curve
5. Coccyx

Figure 125: The spine.

Bibliography

Anatomical Chart Co., Chicago: Muscular System and Skeletal System.

Anderson, B.: 1990. Stretching. Pelham Books, London.

Andrews, E.: 1991. Muscle Management. Thorsons, London.

Barcsay, J.: 1997. Anatomy for the Artist. Black Cat, USA.

Barnard, D.: 2000. The Effect of Passive 'Soft Tissue Release' on Elbow Range of Movement and Spasticity When Applied to the Elbow Flexors and Forearm Supinators of a Hemiplegic Stroke Patient – A Single Case Study. Brighton University.

Butler, D.: 1991. Mobilisation of the Nervous System. Churchill Livingstone, Edinburgh.

Cantu, R. I., Grodin, A. J.: 1992. Myofascial Manipulation – Theory and Clinical Application. Aspen Publishers In., Maryland, USA.

Cantu, R., Grodin, A.: 1992. In: J. DeLany, 'Connective Tissue Perspectives'. *Journal of Bodywork and Movement Therapies*, 4(4) 273–275.

Cash, M.: 1996. Sport and Remedial Massage Therapy. Ebury Press, London.

Chaitow, L.: 1990. Soft Tissue Manipulation. Healing Arts Press, USA.

Chaitow, L.: 1996. Modern Neuromuscular Techniques. Churchill Livingstone, New York.

Commerford, M. J., Mottram, S. L.: 2000. Functional Stability Re-training – Principles and Strategies for Managing Mechanical Dysfunction. *Journal of Manual Therapy*, 6(1) 3–14.

Commerford, M. J., Mottram, S. L.: 2000. Movement and Stability Dysfunction – Contemporary Developments. *Journal of Manual Therapy*, 6(1) 15–26.

Dick, F.: 1992. Sports Training Principles. A & C Black, London.

Gray, H.: 1993. Gray's Anatomy. Magpie Books Ltd.

Grisogono, V.: 1991. Sports Injuries. John Murray, London.

Hemery, D., Ogden, G., Evans, A.: 1991. Winning Without Drugs. Thorsons.

Holey, E. A.: 2000. Connective Tissue Massage – a Bridge Between Complementary and Orthodox Approaches. *Journal of Bodywork and Movement Therapies*, 4(1) 72–80.

Juhan, D.: 1987. In: J. DeLany, 'Connective Tissue Perspectives'. *Journal of Bodywork and Movement Therapies*, 4(4) 273–275, 2000.

Juhan, D.: 1998. Job's Body – A Handbook for Bodywork. Station Hill, Barrytown Limited.

Lederman, E.: 1997. Fundamentals of Manual Therapy: Physiology, Neurology and Psychology. Churchill Livingstone, Edinburgh.

Lowe, W. W.: 1999. Active Engagement Strokes. *Journal of Bodywork and Movement Therapies*, 4(4) 277–278.

McAtee, B.: 1993. Facilitated Stretching. Human Kinetics, USA.

McMinn, R. M. H., Hutchings, R. T., Pegington, J., Abrahams, P. H.: 1993. A Colour Atlas of Human Anatomy. Wolfe, USA.

McMinn, R. M. H., Hutchings, R. T., Logan, B. M.: 1982. Foot and Ankle Anatomy. Wolfe, USA.

Myers, T. W.: 1997. The 'Anatomy Trains'. *Journal of Bodywork and Movement Therapies*, 1(2) 91–101.

Myers, T. W.: 1997. The 'Anatomy Trains', Part 2. *Journal of Bodywork and Movement Therapies*, 1(3) 134–145.

Noakes, T.: 1991. Lore of Running. Leisure Press, USA.

Norris, C. M.: 1993. Sports Injuries: Diagnosis and Management. Butterworth Heinemann, Oxford.

Oschman, J. L.: 1997. What is Healing Energy? Gravity, Structure and Emotions. *Journal of Bodywork and Movement Therapies*, 1(5) 297–309.

Oschman, J. L.: 1997. In J. DeLany, 'Connective Tissue Perspectives'. *Journal of Bodywork and Movement Therapies*, 4(4) 273–275.

Plastanga, N., Field, D., Soames, R.: 1995. Anatomy and Human Movement. Butterworth Heinemann, Oxford.

Read, M., Wade, P.: 1997. Sports Injuries. Butterworth Heinemann, Oxford.

Rolf, I. P.: 1989. Rolfing, 1st edition. Healing Arts Press, USA.

Sperryn, P. N.: 1985. Sport and Medicine. Butterworth Heinemann, Oxford.

Stone, R., Stone, J.: 2001. Atlas of Skeletal Muscles. McGraw Hill, USA.

Tortora and Anagnostakos: 1997. Principles of Anatomy and Physiology, 8th ed. John Wiley & Sons, Chichester.

Williams, D.: 1995. In: J. DeLany, 'Connective Tissue Perspectives'. *Journal of Bodywork and Movement Therapies*, 4(4) 273–275, 2000.

Wilmore, J. H., Costill, D. L.: 1994. Physiology of Sport and Exercise. Human Kinetics, USA.

Wirhed, R.: 1989. Athletic Ability and the Anatomy of Motion. Wolfe, USA.

Ylinen, J. Cash, M.: 1988. Sports Massage. Ebury Press, London.

Index